"An insightful and Helpful Read – A book that provides insight into the thoughts and feelings of a young man with ASD. This book brings more understanding to the complex nature of autism and its impacts on self and immediate family. As an educator, I've seen the observable behavior of children with autism but have never witnessed the inward thoughts and feelings which this book made possible. It brought forth an awareness that as humans we desire to understand and to be understood."

~Laurel Ruddy
Educator—California

"I really enjoyed reading Autism in Hindsight. It was an incredibly moving story. It made me want to learn more about how Isaiah overcame the obstacles of having autism and OCD as an adult. I thought this book was special because it not only captured the journey with Isaiah but also his relationship with his mom."

~Ceejay Washington
Special Education Para-Educator—Iowa

"I found Autism in Hindsight really educational as it introduces the different diagnoses. I think for someone that is looking for answers this is a good step in the right direction. Monica shared her heart as far as facing this in her son's life. Isaiah also shared his inner self as he spoke of the journey that he has. The different situations that happened in his life and how he handled it.

How wonderful that Isaiah wanted to pursue treatment as

an adult. I hope that this book will reach others that have not accepted that they have lived under some kind of disability that could have been set in a direction of a better life.

I enjoyed the book from the standpoint of a mother that has lived with mental illness in the family for most of my life. Our journey has not been as successful as yours."

~Linda Souza
Book Reviewer—California

Before reading *Autism in Hindsight* I had little knowledge of autism, and other issues that it can awaken. It's amazing how far the resources mentioned have come over the last few years. The Q & A format was helpful in following along. My heart appreciated the transparency, honesty, truth and freedom that was spoken between mother and son. No doubt each word written was covered in prayer.

I highly recommend this book to anyone that is a teacher, as well as those that have a friend or family member that is on the spectrum, or could be on the spectrum.

~Annette Medina
Book Reviewer—California

I am so thankful for Monica and Isaiah for sharing their journey. It was so insightful and has helped me understand better the journey those who are on the autism spectrum are experiencing.

~Lynn Orellana
Book Reviewer—California

Autism in Hindsight

also by
Monica Cane

Scrambled Hormones
60 Days of Encouragement
for Moms Raising Teenage Daughters

Autism in Hindsight

A Candid Conversation Between Mother and Son

MONICA CANE

WITH ISAIAH CANE

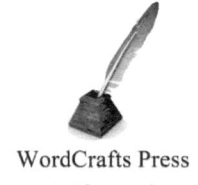

WordCrafts Press

Autism in Hindsight
Copyright © 2024
Monica Cane

ISBN: 978-1-962218-29-0

Cover design by Mike Parker

Published by WordCrafts Press
Cody, Wyoming 82414
www.wordcrafts.net

To all the beautiful diagnosed and undiagnosed
people on the spectrum.
You fit. You're loved. You belong.

Contents

People write for so many different reasons. Some write to share their creative gift of storytelling, some to vent, some as a way to talk to God, others journal to better understand themselves and some write to share their extensive knowledge on fascinating topics of interest. Then there are some people, like myself, who feel a deep need to write for the sake of sharing a bit of their own life journey in hopes of encouraging at least one person, if not more along the way.

Autism in Hindsight is that kind of book. A bit of sharing about my son, Isaiah, and what it was like for him and for us, his parents, to discover that he was autistic. This discovery did not take place as a child, as one might assume, but when Isaiah was eighteen years old. *Autism in Hindsight* shares some of Isaiah's and my thoughts and experiences before, during, and after his diagnosis.

When I first pitched the idea for this book, I considered a couple different ways I could write it; ways that might make it the most marketable. I thought I could detail this experience from my perspective, which tends to be my go to style of writing, but I didn't think that would bring out all that needed to be said. I then considered writing this book in the third-person as a flowing short story to add a little extra spice to draw readers in. Pretty marketable idea right? But that didn't sit right with me either, because in truth I didn't want to *spice* anything up. I want to be authentic, whether marketable or not. In the end, I opted for sharing this part of Isaiah's life-journey and my own as his mama in complete truth and in the style that best reflects how Isaiah and I engage with each other. We talk a lot and ask questions. Okay, maybe I take the lead on that part but together, we share our thoughts honestly. We have great conversations, so that is how this book is written—a genuine conversation between mother and son, asking questions and sharing answers. In it, we dissect some of the good and bad that comes from learning that you are on the Autism spectrum as a young adult, along with other thoughts, feelings, and issues that have come up for each of us along the way. In other words, mother and son are having one of their meaningful chats, and this time we are inviting you in.

With as many fantastic conversations Isaiah and I have had pretty much since the moment he said his first words, I must say our conversations have gotten a whole lot deeper during the last five years as we have learned what being on the spectrum meant, both pre- and post-diagnosis. Although I was there and fully knew my son's story before, during, and after his diagnosis, I wanted to interview him to delve deeper into this part of his life so he could express himself honestly, now that we are a few years into this journey and have some beneficial hindsight.

As I put together my list of questions for Isaiah, I told myself a number of times to make sure to simply listen once the interviewing began. I knew once he started answering questions and reflecting back to when he was younger—when my husband and I had absolutely no clue that autism was even something to consider—there might be some things he would say that would make me sad or angry or feel some sort of way as a mama. Even more so because I was such a helicopter mom who took pride in over-anticipating all of my children's thoughts, needs, and feelings. I knew there would be a chance during our question and answer time that I would want to defend myself as a parent, but I also knew it wouldn't be necessary. Isaiah has his own perspective, and I really do value it. I have my own perspective, and thankfully, my son values mine as well.

This book is divided into four sections. The first three sections cover Isaiah's initial diagnosis and then others, along with his choice to confront fears and the process of finding himself. In the beginning of these sections, I share a bit of my own viewpoint of that particular season of life before I go on to ask Isaiah a handful of questions based on what I observed to be relevant at the time. In truth, these questions only briefly describe his experiences, but they do give insight to the challenges he faced as he has learned to navigate his world through the lens of autism. At the end of each section, I share a few final words; first, to emphasize the advantage of hindsight, but mostly I share final words because moms always want to have the last word whether they are having a personal conversation or writing a book with their adult child.

As for the fourth and final section of this book, interestingly enough, it was a dear friend of mine who encouraged me to flip the format. Sharing with her the idea for the book, I explained that I would be asking Isaiah dozens of questions about being on the spectrum and giving him the opportunity to share his experience. She loved the idea and then added, *Perhaps Isaiah can interview you as well.*

My immediate reaction was, *Why?* I didn't think there would be anything Isaiah would want to know about me in regards to my perspective on this subject that he didn't already know. But the more I considered the idea, the more

I began to wonder, *What kind of questions would Isaiah think to ask, if given the opportunity?*

Eventually I decided to just ask Isaiah if he would even be interested in something like that, and when I did, he was quick to respond with an enthusiastic, *Yes!* I gave him free reign to get his list together and ask whatever questions he had on his mind. I wasn't sure what direction he would go with his questions, but since our goal with this book was honest conversation, I thought, *Let's do it!* I was surprised, yet perhaps not all that surprised, by the questions he chose. They were questions I believe he wanted and perhaps needed to ask to get to know me, his mama, even better as a human being.

Being such a niche book where we share our personal experience with the autism spectrum in the context of hindsight, has caused me to think about who might pick this book up to read it—other than curious friends and family members. Ultimately, I wondered who would truly benefit from this book? After giving much thought to the question, I concluded that anyone who picks up this book can benefit in some manner. Whether it's learning about autism for the first time, seeing what the spectrum looks like through Isaiah's eyes, or recognizing the value of being fully aware of your own mental health needs, I believe this book has something for whoever chooses to read it.

If nothing else, my hope and prayer for this book is that it will encourage readers to be brave and have candid conversations about those really tough issues, about those things they are uncomfortable with, or like me—maybe missed along the way. Whether it's about disorders, disabilities, mental health issues, or just funky family stuff, if our conversation in this book encourages readers to have honest conversations without judgment with the ones they love, then it is well worth it.

With that said, let me tell how it began.

"If you've met one person with autism, you've met one person with autism."

–Dr. Stephen Shore

I had been in a deep sleep for a few hours when I found myself slowly waking up to the sound of muffled voices. Trying to clear the cobwebs from my sleepy brain, I strained my ear to see if I could figure out who was talking. It had to be close to midnight, so I couldn't imagine who would be calling let alone visiting at that time. As I became more fully awake, I listened more intently and felt fairly certain I was hearing my son talking to someone. Whoever it was seemed to have a higher pitched voice. I thought perhaps it was a girl. But who? What girl? At eighteen years old, Isaiah was still pretty shy; he didn't really talk to too many girls, so who the heck was on the other side of my bedroom door talking to my son? That question became more prominent in my mind and caused me to sit up straight in bed, clear my head, and listen with intent to figure out who the mystery guest was. I don't recall the words of the conversation, but I distinctly heard two different voices. It took a few more minutes of intent listening—and then suddenly, I knew.

My son was carrying on both sides of the conversation. It was indeed a dialogue between two people, but he was playing both characters. When I realized my son was having a full-blown conversation with himself and talking in different voices, I felt scared. Not *of* him, but *for* him.

I had heard Isaiah talk aloud to himself many times prior and had never felt concern. As a matter of fact, I often talk aloud to myself when writing, working, or taking in some sort of information. Talking out loud just helps me process whatever it is I'm trying to do. Because studies show that talking out loud helps us organize our thoughts, whenever I talked out loud to myself or overheard Isaiah doing the same, I wasn't concerned in any way.

Until that night.

That night was different.

As concern for my son overwhelmed me, I started praying. *Is something wrong with my son, God? Is he alright? Please help him. Let me know what to do.*

I didn't want to go into the kitchen and alarm or embarrass Isaiah at that moment, but I knew in the morning we would need to have a serious talk.

It was difficult to fall back to sleep, but I eventually did. The next day I sat down with Isaiah and shared my concerns about hearing him talking to himself in the middle of the night. I don't recall exactly what he said, but I sure do remember the look on his face. Before speaking to him, I had been so worried that I might embarrass him or hurt his feelings in some way. But embarrassment or hurt was not the look he gave me. It was more...non-reactive. His look seemed to say, *This is my norm. What are you so worried about?*

I was grateful not to witness hurt in his eyes, but I also wasn't sure what to do with the, *This is my norm,* look he gave. We talked a bit more, and I went on to suggest he consider speaking to a counselor—just to air out his thoughts and feelings. I'm not fully sure if in that moment Isaiah was just being a good, compliant son or if he really saw the value of connecting with a counselor based on my concern, but either way he agreed without hesitation.

Around the time Isaiah was making arrangements to see a counselor, I happened to be listening to the Ted Talk App

I had recently downloaded on my phone. This was a couple years before discovering TikTok influencer and content creator Corey Singer, but similarly, videos would pop up on my Ted Talk feed, and I would listen to many of them, no matter the subject. Up to this point, I had never heard of Asperger's, so I wasn't seeking out specific videos on the subject, but somehow, one day, *My Life with Asperger's* by Daniel Wendler popped up. I listened to Daniel's Ted Talk and then listened to it again. Something was there. Something was clicking in mind. It wasn't one specific thing he said, I think it was just all of it. Something about Daniel's life with Asperger's caused me to significantly pause and wonder about this thing called Asperger's, and if it could possibly relate to my son.

Shortly after, I told Isaiah how I had come across the video and explained that while I could be completely wrong, I was recognizing some sort of connection between him and the things Daniel Wendler said about Asperger's. I suggested that Isaiah talk to his counselor about it to see if there might be anything there. Fortunately, he thought it was a good idea as well and brought the question to his counselor. And so it began.

As Isaiah explains throughout this book, he went to a few different counselors before settling in more permanently with one counselor he really connected with, but with each initial counselor he saw, he told them what he had been experiencing, and they all seemed to come to the same conclusion. The consensus was that Isaiah was very likely somewhere on the spectrum.

How strange it all was for me. I had known my son his entire life. I raised him, and while I did notice a few little quirks, there was nothing out of the ordinary. As a matter of fact I tended to agree with all of his teachers who felt that Isaiah was wise beyond his years and highly intelligent. Naturally, I'm a bit biased because he is my son, but he just seemed like a lovely little grown up right from the start. Even if there was something quirky from time to time, it didn't faze me, because grown-ups and little grown-ups are all kind of quirky in my opinion. But as Isaiah met with a variety of trained professionals, all of them seemed to clearly see what we had never seen before.

While I'm not one to automatically believe the first thing someone tells me about one of my children, being that we were starting to hear the same thing over and over about the spectrum as it related to Isaiah, we concluded that it was valid, and that we needed to learn about what it was *exactly*, how it was affecting Isaiah, and how we could help.

Honestly, the biggest help in our understanding came from Isaiah himself. He was eighteen when he received his diagnosis and legally considered an adult. I couldn't badger the counselors for information—though I would have if I could have. I had to either rely on what the research told us about being on the spectrum, which I quickly learned didn't mean it all applied to my son, or I could wait and see if Isaiah would be willing to explain what was going on and teach us from his perspective. Fortunately, teaching mom and dad was right up Isaiah's alley. In the last few years, Isaiah has been able to clearly articulate the differences and/or similarities between what studies reveal about someone on the spectrum and what he personally experiences.

Initially, it was all so shocking and eye-opening, in hindsight, the dots continue to connect. At first, there was a strong temptation for self-condemnation for not recognizing something sooner. Thankfully, God reminded me that self-condemnation never gets you anywhere. The truth is, the spectrum is broad and ever-evolving, and there's still a lot to learn, so instead of condemnation, we do our best to stay open to understanding.

For the Lord gives wisdom;
from his mouth comes knowledge
and understanding.

–Proverbs 2:6

Part I

I confess, I have been a bit obsessed with TikTok, the social media platform where people from all over the world create every type of short video that you can imagine. Anything from singing, dancing, painting, comedy skits, recipes, how-to-tips and tricks, funny pet adventures, never seen before movie bloopers, and so much more. Ever since the world shut down in March of 2020, TikTok with its quick fifteen seconds all the way up to ten minute video clips has been a fantastic source of entertainment for me and for the over 1.53 billion other users around the world.

When I first started skimming through the creative videos, apparently I was clicking "like" on a lot of slapstick humor because my *For You* page was flooded with them. For the one or two people who may be unfamiliar with TikTok, a *For You* page is generated by TikTok's algorithms, allowing the App to push more videos that you seem to like in your direction. Interestingly enough, in the midst of all the crazy, silly, slapstick skits flooding my *For You* page, an unexpected video by a content creator named Cory Singer @thecorysinger happened to pop up on my feed. Though I had no idea who he was or why he ended up on my page, I thought I would give his video a try because his warm smile led me to believe he was probably a nice guy, so why not listen to what he had to say? From the very moment he started speaking, I was hooked, because he was telling his viewers what it was like having Asperger's.

It hadn't been all that long since my son had been diagnosed with Asperger's and we were still learning what exactly that meant. So here was this adorable guy, Cory, just casually talking about his experiences and letting viewers into his world. He spoke about the good, the bad and the very misunderstood aspects of Asperger's.

Through some previous research I had learned a little bit, but I didn't know anyone else with Asperger's—I just knew my son. I began scrolling through other video's Cory had and just felt an odd sense of connection. I eventually found one video where Cory explained the meaning of the word "Masking" which is when someone learns, practices, and performs certain behaviors and suppresses others in order to be more like the people around them. It was the first time I had actually heard of the word, but as soon as Cory described what it looked like for him and how exhausting it all was, I was immediately able to recognize it was something I had seen in my son.

After clicking "like" on pretty much every video Cory made, the algorithms began pushing other videos having to do with autism onto my feed. Many of these videos were made by parents of young autistic children who were making strides in their own understanding while learning how to best help their child navigate the world through an autistic lens. Isaiah did not necessarily display the same symptoms as many of the videos I watched, other than the ones I saw of Cory's. However, there was something there that clicked for me. It was through these many videos that I was able to learn about this very unfamiliar thing called "being on the spectrum" and how varied the spectrum really is.

I remember when Isaiah first received the diagnosis of Asperger's, I thought it was just this one particular thing and that I needed to find answers in order to best help my son. The challenging part however is that when your child is eighteen years old when he gets a diagnosis like this—or any other for that matter—you can only go so far in helping because at that point he is considered an adult and has to be the one calling the shots.

In other words, mommy can't be calling all the doctors to speak on her adult baby's behalf, demanding answers or finding out exactly how the conversation went down with the diagnosing counselor and if there was any pertinent information missed along the way.

All those little details that mamas of children under eighteen would be allowed to control, I really couldn't. Sure, I could find *some* information through research, but really, it was up to my adult son.

Ultimately, I had to just walk side-by-side with him while he took the lead in pursuing help and understanding of his own mental health. Fortunately, Isaiah cared about his own wellbeing and was willing to learn about Asperger's and his overall mental health. He was also willing to let me be a part of the process as much as I was able.

For the first two years after his initial diagnosis, it seemed to me that every time we would gain a little momentum in understanding what it all meant, a new layer of symptoms or issues were uncovered, revealing there was more there than met the eye.

We began to realize that this "one Asperger thing" wasn't just one thing at all. It was connected to being autistic, which in turn had a common comorbidity with Obsessive Compulsive Disorder (OCD) along with anxiety and low self esteem and more. As layers were uncovered we began to grasp just how broad and definite the autism spectrum is.

I admit, I found it difficult to completely wrap my head around Isaiah being on the spectrum for two reasons. One being that my understanding of autism, if at all, was that someone would show disabilities and be most likely be non-verbal from birth. In other words, I wholeheartedly assumed if someone was autistic, you would recognize it a mile away. Because this was my basic understanding, the second reason I couldn't wrap my head around it all is because Isaiah showed no signs whatsoever when he was little. What he did show was that he was an extremely sweet natured, very intelligent little boy. He excelled in school, he was a part of student council, and at the recommendation of his teachers, he participated in the G.A.T.E Program *(Gifted and Talented Education)* and was also a peer tutor. These were not things that I would have associated with someone who was on the spectrum. From our very limited viewpoint as parents in regard to autism, along with the view of his educators, Martial Arts instructor, and pretty much every adult Isaiah engaged with, he was simply considered a kind, sweet, and super-smart kid.

The only thing I ever noticed as perhaps different when Isaiah was little was that he often thought other boys his age were immature. With the exception of two boys that I can recall, both who were also considered highly intelligent, Isaiah just wasn't all that interested in spending time with other kids his age. Honestly, he seemed to prefer talking to adults more than his peers. But I never thought much of it. I actually thought it was kind of cute. Then again, as a completely biased mama, I thought everything he did, along with his two sisters when they all were little, was pretty darn cute.

Looking back, I now find it strange how you can view

things one way for so long and be so certain that your views are correct and then something happens that causes your view to change. It wasn't until Isaiah was eighteen years old and I began noticing he was talking to himself in a different sort of way that my view started to change. Could there be something different going on that I, the mama who believes she knows all things when it comes to her precious children, never noticed? I'm not going to lie, having to ask yourself that question is a strange and uncomfortable place to be.

As uncomfortable as that time was, I'm grateful for it. I'm thankful for uncovering layers upon layers of unknown things because it not only allowed us to discover Isaiah was on the spectrum, but it opened a proverbial can of worms that started us on a road to honest communication and healing that I didn't fully realize we needed.

*"Autism can't define me,
I define autism."*

–Dr. Kerry Magro

Talking with Isaiah

When did you first notice differences between you and your peers, and what specifically had you noticed?

I didn't have a lot of space for comparison between myself and my peers when I was young, because I was homeschooled from sixth through tenth grade. However, when I was in fifth grade, I did notice some divergence. I found myself irritated with kids my age because I was much more task oriented and *people pleasy*. As someone who was extremely task oriented, it was a big deal for me to get specific things done in a timely manner. Usually those specific things were whatever the teacher wanted, and I definitely wanted to please the teacher. So when I started to recognize that most of my peers were not as focused on getting tasks done and pleasing the teacher the way I was, they became a real nuisance to me.

Everyone has natural personality quirks like wanting to be extra organized and being task oriented in general, but years later I learned that my *need* to accomplish a set goal and my frustration with others who were not on the same page was definitely amplified by the fact that I am autistic.

Even now as an adult, getting a task done and wanting it to be done correctly is still something I get frustrated with at times. For example, if someone can't process the need to be on time when I've said something is important, it frustrates me because I'm still seeking to accomplish something specific. No matter my relation to the person, I'm trying to accomplish a goal, and it makes me not want to have that goal in the first place if they are going to rupture that attempt.

It absolutely can still be a challenge for me, but I am learning better ways of coping with it now.

Prior to getting diagnosed as autistic, was there anyone or anything that caught your attention as seeming similar to how you actually felt?

When I was homeschooled I would listen to church sermons on my computer because I identified with the sense of wanting vitality and encouragement, but I really couldn't put my finger on it or identify with exactly what I needed. It crossed my mind that maybe my self-esteem needed to be built up, but I just didn't know why. All I knew was that I had the desire to receive encouragement in a way that I could understand. I found it in a variety of people online and would play their messages, sermons, and podcasts in the background on my computer while doing my school work.

Then there was a TV show that ran for years that I started watching, called *Monk*. It was kind of a quirky, gimmicky show about a detective with Obsessive–Compulsive Disorder (OCD). Looking back, the show isn't the most realistic, but it was something I identified with in terms of feeling shrouded by uncertainty and feeling inappropriate to my environment. I was always trying to better understand what was around me and trying to feel safe, not in a physical sense, but emotionally. I think the character of Monk resonated with me a lot without even knowing it at the time because as an autistic person it's easy to become extremely interested in one thing and hyper-fixate. So for me, identifying with Monk's many fears and feelings of uncertainty made it super easy for me to become hyper-fixated on the show. Even though I couldn't connect the dots yet, *Monk* was a source of comfort for me, especially at the time when I didn't have much of a life outside of school.

I studied Martial Arts for six years, but at a certain point after starting homeschool, I decided to stop pursuing Martial Arts as it wasn't really an emotionally healthy thing for me anymore. I constantly felt like I wasn't good enough with the instructor I had. So I focused on school and would spend thirteen to fourteen hours a day on schoolwork. I didn't realize I had OCD at the time, but there is one specific OCD theme called, "Just Right OCD," which is where a person will do the same thing over and over until it is "just right." If they don't get things just right they can feel as if something terrible will happen. It's similar to that irrational thought, *If you step on a crack, you'll break your mother's back,* but taken literally. When you have OCD, you have the mental capacity to know it's irrational but it still *feels* very real. There were times that I felt if I didn't do the thirteen hours of schoolwork to get it just right, that something awful would happen. I would fail the assignment, or I wouldn't go past the grade I was in, etc. Since it seemed to me that every authority figure, from teachers, to parents, and even my Martial Arts instructor expected me to do well in school, school became the biggest thing for me and the biggest threat to fail in.

You didn't suspect that you were autistic or had OCD, so what led you to the point of wanting to meet with a counselor?

Actually, it was when you, my mom, noticed that I seemed to be mumbling and talking aloud to myself more than usual.

For me at the time, thinking and talking out loud was a gentle dissociative thing that I didn't even think twice about. It was a way to ensure I had company that I enjoyed, because that wasn't always a guarantee. At times I felt bored and wanted company, but at the same time, I was anxious and didn't want to socialize. If I did make any small attempt to actually socialize it was usually in a structured environment like in the classroom or during Martial Arts class where instructors controlled the overall dynamic, and because of that, it didn't feel like a friendship could truly flourish in a way that was comfortable for me. At that age, I didn't have a sense of autonomy as I was rather sheltered under my parents' wings. Even though it was done in a very nice sense, I don't think I was challenged enough to seek my own betterment. On top of that, dealing with OCD and being on the spectrum without knowing it made it even harder. So, yeah, talking to myself was something I felt I did because I was more comfortable stimulating myself with different thoughts, ideas, and conversation, but at a certain point it became a concern for my mom, so I decided to see a counselor.

How did the autism diagnosis come about when you started counseling?

I bounced between a few different counselors before settling in with one. When I talked to one of the first counselors, I was happy about it because I did feel like I had some things emotionally I needed to unfurl. As we began to talk, it occurred to the counselor that I might be autistic just from the very broadly-known traits, such as discomfort with socializing, high intelligence, special interests, and hyper-fixation.

All those things started to paint a picture of potential autism. Unfortunately this counselor moved out of state within only a few months of speaking with him. It's always awkward to put yourself out there in any sense, especially when you are seeking any sort of psychological help, so I took some time before finding another counselor.

I eventually found another counselor I talked to for a bit before mentioning that my mom had found an article on autism and noticed I had a lot of the symptoms. The counselor went into greater depth about autism and explained how symptoms can vary. It was nice for me to finally get some sort of understanding. The counselor said she was going to do a formal assessment, but so many things got switched around in her schedule that we just ended up talking over a period of sessions. By the time it came around to doing anything formal, we both already knew. I was on the spectrum.

As far as formal testing goes, it really consisted of her searching through a Diagnostic and Statistical Manual (DSM 5), which is basically a psychological dictionary that gives the symptoms of every disorder you can think of. It is the same manual a psychiatrist used when I went to him months later about possibly needing medication for anxiety. The psychiatrist asked about my autism diagnosis and agreed with it. From there, we started talking at great lengths about the anxiety I was now experiencing, and based on his assessment, I was also diagnosed with OCD.

As my psychiatrist prescribed medication for OCD, I connected with a few other counselors who all agreed with both diagnoses. Some of the counselors identified it as Asperger's while others said it was Autistic Spectrum Disorder (ASD). There is no difference between Asperger's and ASD really, the only reason they call them different things is the terminology in terms of what is considered most appropriate or sensitive to a group of people. ASD is more of an emerging descriptor because it's hard to categorize a lot of behaviors into a box, especially when it varies between male and female patients, as well as the fact that things may change as people get older. While Asperger's is no longer a term typically used, the symptoms and every trait associated with Asperger's is on the autism spectrum. While OCD is its own phenomenon, research does suggest that autistic people are more likely to experience it, though it has nothing directly to do with the spectrum.

Can you describe the spectrum in layman's terms?

I remember you, Mom, asking the psychiatrist if there was a number that could explain where I was at on the spectrum, and he went on to explain how there is no number, or numerical order, because the spectrum is not a straight line. It's like doing art on an iPad. There is a whole wheel of colors to choose from. The colors don't stand alone; they slowly blend into each other with no real beginning or end, and they just kind of keep going. That's autism.

You don't have a number scale that shows you're a nine out of ten autistic. That's not how it works, but that's how a lot of people picture it. Much more realistically, you just experience your symptoms and they can vary quite a bit. Some people show mild symptoms in some areas. Such as they have no hyper-fixation, but they're completely non-verbal, which is considered a more severe symptom. Others are highly verbal, but they have intense fears that they don't know how to articulate. They can speak well, but they don't have the emotional tools. That was the basis that went along with every autism diagnosis I had. I was told, "you are a capable person, you just don't have the tools to express yourself in conventional forms." So being on the spectrum could mean you are socially awkward and don't know how to relate your feelings that you feel deeply to other people, or perhaps you are non-verbal and can't relate those feelings because your brain can't execute the processes necessary in order to share your feelings. This is the base that ties all of the autism spectrum together.

How did you feel when you first received the diagnosis?

It made me feel seen. A lot of people with autism struggle with self esteem because they don't feel like they are in their element, so they are having to adapt to a situation or environment that they are not comfortable in. Those awkward feelings really kind of wreck your self esteem in addition to anything else that might naturally affect your self esteem as a person. Getting diagnosed as autistic did help to feel some semblance of self esteem, some semblance of belonging. Not to a group or to a group identity but just a competency as a person. It was like finally recognizing that you are a different take, a genetic remix so to speak, but you exist, it's valid, and you are not alone in what you are experiencing. Being seen was not only the effect but the desired effect. It wasn't about getting some autism medication, which there is none of course. It was a matter of contextualizing my experience and validating it, and when that happened, it felt good to be seen.

From there, I didn't know what I wanted because I was still trying to process information. As I continued on with counseling I would just talk about whatever I was feeling, or any issues I was having, but now the counselor was able to incorporate the lens of, "now that we know you are autistic, this may be a new way to see this situation and to better understand yourself."

Do You have an example of incorporating this lens that you can share?

When I was seeing one counselor, I told her there was a girl I liked, and I was scared out of my mind to talk to her. On the surface, that is a very normal teenage thing. However, as I went into detail about how much I would have to plan any conversation I would have, how I would have to script it, rehearse, predetermine my body language, and prepare myself to act normal because I felt fundamentally inferior to others, but especially the girl, my counselor was able to explain what was likely going on for me as an autistic person. She explained to me that I was "masking," trying to mimic the intricacies of perceived normal behavior. She said it is very common and very exhausting for autistic people. I had been trying so hard to act like a normal human being in order to make a good impression, but when the counselor explained this, it changed the context completely for me. I realized for the first time, *Oh I don't have to do this. This is not some objectively necessary thing, this is something I am choosing to do, something I'm forcing myself into.* It helped me a lot to finally have this understanding.

Difficulty developing or maintaining close relationships is one of the symptoms associated with autism. Since masking was an issue in regards to connecting with people, was it always hard developing friendships for you?

I think a lot of people struggle with the desire for friends, but as I got older, I think the struggle turned into disinterest. Being autistic, whether before or after getting diagnosed, I had more of a, meet-me-where-I'm-at mindset. I was interested in knowing someone who honestly shared my interests and personality type, versus just having a bunch of people around to call friends.

That is the ideology for a lot of people who are autistic, where we don't want to be flexible with much, but we want to meet someone who happens to be in our lane, whether it be co-workers, friends, or dating. When you do find a person in your lane, it makes you feel like you can *finally* relate to someone, which is a huge deal. For me, it was a labor to relate to co-workers or individuals in formal settings, because I felt they were either very boring, or I didn't share their motivations. When I was young, I just couldn't understand the fascination with girls, guns, and trucks that most guys seemed to have. I just didn't feel the same way. Maybe my perception is warped due to social media, but a lot of people my age just seemed very involved with themselves and needed public and open praise, and that wasn't for me. I was more classically co-dependent and wanted private and personal praise to feel like I was enough.

The possibility of friendship became a little easier when I started working for a congressional campaign. It created a sort of natural bond because we all had a shared goal, so conversations became easier at work and outside of work. We were getting to know each other on a personal level without anything being forced or feeling like you have to do that thing that autistic people dread—put yourself out there and try to socialize because someone else insists.

I've definitely come to understand that when I do things I'm passionate about, it's much easier for me to make friends. For example, when I have anything to do with screenwriting, it is so much easier to socialize with someone of kindred interests, because I don't feel tempted to modify my behavior.

The same applies in dating, really. I mean if I can't connect with a girl because she's just too into herself and we share no common goals, I wouldn't feel an attraction, and I'm not going to want to know more about her. What initially caught my attention when I first met my girlfriend wasn't anything to do with race, appearance, or socioeconomic status; she just had a beautifully similar sense of humor, and that stayed with me. It had more staying power than any vanity attempts to impress me would have. Humor and shared interests gave me a sense of security and comfort. It was inviting. It influenced a degree of commonality, not just having something in common but having something in common that we both *chose*, like prioritizing interpersonal connections, prioritizing empathic work ethics, and learning how best to help those around us. Connecting on that level is hard for people in general, and even more so when you're autistic. Fortunately, she was able to meet me where I was, and I happily did the same with her.

After learning you were autistic and had OCD, you then learned that you had codependent tendencies. How did that discovery come about?

Being codependent wasn't something I realized was a thing. It was normal for me. I thought that was just how people were. I only started recognizing codependency as a potentially negative trait in my first relationship. I was having a conversation with my girlfriend at the time, and she said, "I can't be okay unless you're okay." I later re-encountered that phrase as the exact definition of codependency in the book *Codependent No More* by Melody Beattie.

Through that relationship, I learned how a codependent person operates. Hearing her say that simple and clear phrase, "I can't be okay unless you're okay," about me as well as her family members really made it click for me. I thought, *I've clearly experienced that. That is what I've felt most of my life.*

It's difficult because codependency exists in a different sector of human behavior than autism and OCD, which are both almost strictly seen on a neurological level. Those are things you can identify early on. You may not detect them at first, but the differences in the brain are there and are notable. Codependency is something that is developed, something that is taught by experiences, it's extremely trauma-informed.

I know people try to centralize blame on their parents in regards to their issues, but it really wasn't just with my parents. It was a combination of factors which was compounded by seeing it all through the lens of autism. Still, there definitely was a codependent dynamic in my family. When you are a child, you are naturally weaker physically and emotionally, so you depend on the people around you and want to keep them happy. There is an interdependence, a reliance, which is perfectly fine, but codependence, where you think, *I can't be okay unless you are okay,* can be kind of an emotional survival tool. That's how it felt for me but I didn't realize that's what it was until seeing it in someone else. That short-lived relationship with my ex really opened my eyes to my own codependent nature and made me scrounge below the surface.

When I was at a young impressionable age, there was a lot of tension between my mom and one of my sisters. She was an exceptionally rebellious teen, and my mom was very fearful that the lifestyle she was living would end badly. My mom had her own struggle with codependency which she herself didn't realize, yet revealed itself a lot in the struggles she had with my sister.

I often felt scared and anxious whenever I would hear yelling or arguing. There was always so much uncertainty in the air. Observing both steadfast codependency from my mom and capricious rebellion from my sister during those turbulent years had a major impact on me.

While having autism made it difficult to express thoughts and feelings in general during that time, having a codependent dynamic within my family added to the difficulties and caused me to adopt those very same tendencies which I believed was normal for everyone. I felt responsible for other people's feelings. Whether it was my parents, my sister, my Martial Arts instructor, or my teachers, I felt responsible. I desperately worked to please them, to the point of ignoring how I felt, which is codependency at its core.

There are definitely overlaps to be had with autism and codependency, but I wouldn't say that one solely caused the other. Part of it was learned by observing it, but a huge part I think was also from the praise I got from being codependent in general, because when you anticipate someone's needs they are typically enthused. In the autistic brain, you especially associate that praise as being an absolutely good thing, so the

31

cycle of anticipating someone's needs and receiving praise continues as codependent nature.

Prior to you getting diagnosed, as your mother I was under the impression that every struggle you had was based on those turbulent years of observing codependency within the family, but it wasn't just that, was it?

It's understandable that you felt that way. And I remember suspecting that was how you felt when we went to a book store and I asked for a book on psychology simply because I was interested, and you immediately asked if I was interested in the book because I wanted to understand the conflict you and my sister were having at the time.

Don't get me wrong, that period was an extremely potent vessel of a lot of communicative traumas that were probably the very core of why I struggled the most. Nevertheless, I was born with autism, and the symptoms began to show as I got older. It's the same way you can have shingles or certain types of cancers but symptoms won't show for years. It's a similar thing with autism, and it absolutely influenced my familial trauma situation.

I don't believe having OCD influenced things much in this area. The OCD, as far back as I can remember, never involved any family issues in terms of any themes. It was just something I was likely to have regardless. Even if I had a tranquil childhood, I would have still had it, but I most likely would have had much better skills for coping. I wouldn't have had to go through as much pain in discovering my OCD and managing it. A lot of what I experience now is not necessarily *bad* but a culmination of messiness. It's not a very reasonable thing to say something like, 'I was around a sibling who got in trouble a lot so that caused everything wrong in the world.' It's more reasonable to say, 'I was around a sibling who got in trouble a lot, *and* I was born autistic, *and* symptoms started to show a little after she left the house, *and* I then started to get symptoms of OCD popping up. Then, when I started therapy, I began to recognize how all these things from childhood had influenced it.' It's not really a straight line.

It's like a bunch of extension cords in a bundle that you're slowly pulling out, and as you do so, one knot unravels without event, and another binds tighter. All these connections are being made. I began to see how different things influenced why I felt like I couldn't express myself or why the person I chose for my first relationship was such an unhealthy person. She rewarded the very negative behaviors that I didn't realize were negative and had been normal up to that point for me.

Not to devalue their trauma via comparison, but it's similar to how kids who were victims of sexual assault are the most likely to end up with abusive partners. Not because they like it, but because it's what their personality naturally draws to. They will naturally go for someone who wows them, and leads this love-bombing stage of providing way too much unhealthy love and affection and then suddenly takes it away. Then teases it and takes it away again, until they just *have* you. You *learn* these relationship traits whether it be from someone who is malicious or just people trying to do their best, which is more often the case.

I have heard you compare codependency as a hamster and OCD/autism as a hamster wheel. Can you explain what that means?

It's the most random but sincere comparison that I can make. I feel like a big overlap between codependency and autism for me is consistently seeking some form of stimulation. I like to feel occupied, as if I am consistently achieving something. Some comedian made a joke about how rodents always seem manic or neurotic no matter what they're doing, and for whatever reason that stuck with me. Being hyper-vigilant to an extent, there's some ironic appeal to trying to complete a task that can only be completed in increments, but never as a whole; temporary satisfaction without a long-term resolution. Developing symptoms of OCD finally provided the missing piece of a self-perpetuating of unhealthy behaviors—or the hamster wheel. Seeking to people-please and hide from my chronic fears made for constant short term rewards. It felt fantastic evading my fears and making someone else happy by undermining myself at times, but I wasn't really solving the larger problems, so the wheel kept coming around. At times, the cycle was exhilarating, as it kept me busy and away from my own feelings. Nonetheless, exhaustion was inevitable for me.

Then there is OCD and autism, that combo emphasizes the brain's capacity to obsess or hyper-fixate on something like fitting in. And suddenly you're in this loop of constantly examining how you are doing, how you think others perceive you, fearing that you might say something inappropriate which eventually leads to hyper-fixating on people pleasing. The trick is when nothing bad happens during an experience, my brain credits that to me being hyper-vigilant; not to me simply being competent. Once someone like myself reaches the people pleasing mode, I'm falsely pleasing three different areas of myself. The OCD part of me is saying, *Oh good, I didn't offend anyone.* The autistic side is saying, *Yay, I can seem like a normal person,* while the Codependent part believes, *They like me, which means I'm worth something.* Momentarily, I might feel like I found what I am looking for. However, the problem is those three areas don't stay relieved, they *always* want more. So they are on that hamster wheel, and they're always gonna keep running because that's what hamster wheels do, they keep coming back around and around until you do something to stop it.

What were some of the greatest takeaways or even hindrances for you as you began to learn more about your diagnosis?

I initially did some degree of research on autism after my diagnosis, but not as much as I did when I got diagnosed with OCD as that was something specific I wanted to resolve. With autism it was just a matter of experiencing congruence between the person I am, the person I want to be, and the person I present myself as. Slowly merging those identities, getting comfortable being myself and asserting myself is a whole hurdle in itself. As I'm slowly honing in on that identity of what I want, it's a matter of understanding what things might be influenced by me being autistic. Like, is this why I hate breaking even the smallest of commitments? Or why I don't like crowds at certain times? Or why I can't stand certain textures of things?

I had no idea that sensory stimulation was a thing until one counselor was doing an assessment and asked me if I had any sensory sensitivities, such as fabrics I really didn't like, or any smells that I couldn't stand? I really didn't know what was exceptional or different from the average person because I had only been in my own body, so to me it was all normal, but I began to learn that for other people it's not. So one of the great takeaways is that as I was slowly able to piece things together in understanding myself, I was able to know what I appreciated and what I could improve on.

On the flip side, as I kind of got the wheels spinning trying to understand myself, I started feeling a lot more feelings, including those which I didn't like, that frightened me but were unrealistic. Thoughts and feelings only after years of running from them would I discover it was a tell-tale sign of OCD.

Prior to my initial diagnosis, my feelings were not my concern or my priority. It was just a matter of staying within certain emotional bounds. I think because I was trying to stay emotionally safe, I ended up trying to contain my feelings by keeping them in a box. That went on for a long time, especially when I was homeschooled. I would have a task at hand and just focus on that. It allowed me to escape from my own feelings. Then in my junior year of high-school I went back to school in-person, where it seemed like containing my feelings were a matter of survival for me because I felt so ill-equipped for social situations.

I attended a different, larger school for my final year of high school. Still unaware of my diagnosis, I was consumed with thinking that I was going to get straight D's because I naturally felt ill-equipped in my environment, and I didn't have self esteem to think I could do it. As it turned out, I ended up getting almost all A's and being fairly well liked. I was surprised by my own performance. Since I didn't feel comfortable, I naturally thought I could not do well, and that crucial misunderstanding, *I don't feel comfortable, I can't do well*, was what guided me through a lot of my emotions.

By the time I began college, I had been diagnosed but knew very little about autism and myself. It was somewhere around that time that I was having constant intrusive images in my head of driving to class, veering off the freeway and crashing with the all-consuming question of *what if I die?* When I relayed this to a particular counselor I was seeing at the time, I don't think he was properly trained enough in OCD because his response began and ended at, "It's normal for people to wonder, *what if?*" My primary physician said the same thing when I relayed my thoughts to him.

I was developing so much stress over these constant *what ifs*, that I was just looking forward to sleeping so I wouldn't have to wake up to the constant *what if?, what if?, what if?.* I was extremely anxious. The thought of killing myself was unrelenting and left me without a moment to think or feel anything else. That type of stuff was occurring and no one had a full answer for it until I connected with a psychiatrist who thankfully had training in regards to OCD.

OCD often gets misdiagnosed as general anxiety because being poorly informed makes the latter an easier diagnosis. These intrusive thoughts came and went in waves for months. I was nineteen when I got diagnosed with OCD, and that was the first time I felt so much pressure just leave me. I vividly recall how the psychiatrist, in the most glib way possible, said, "Oh you just have OCD." Meanwhile, I'm sitting there, a blubbering mess, deathly convinced I won't see twenty-two.

I came to understand that the fundamental mechanism in the brain is the base of your brain, called the amygdala, or what people jokingly refer to as the 'lizard brain' because it's the part we share with lizards. And for lack of better words, it's the stupid part of your brain that develops first. This stupid part of the brain gets first dibs on every thought and emotion you have. It starts at the very center of the brain. The front of the brain, just behind your forehead is called the prefrontal cortex, that's the smart part and the last part to develop. The smart part evolves all the way until you are twenty-five. It's in charge of impulse control, rational thinking, and processing language. Usually, the standard human brain lets the amygdala and frontal cortex communicate. The OCD brain doesn't.

When you have a fear or severe anxiety and it's irrational, if you're a normal person, you think that it's scary but eventually your prefrontal cortex is going to tell your amygdala, *Don't worry about it, I thought about it and turns out that's not a threat.* With OCD, that communication never completes, it's a series of electrical signals that your brain never sends because the neural pathways are inhibited, so you have to kinda tough it out. The amygdala, in charge of processing emotions, survival instincts, and memory, will send stress signals that can save you if you're actually in danger. However, those neural pathways that normally help you relax are blocked, you are in continual stress mode. You are always in fight or flight because you're mis-identifying things as threats. You may see Joe Blow from the grocery store with a box cutter in his hand because he needs to open boxes, but if you're me with OCD, you think, *what if I grab his box cutter and cut my own throat?* That smart part of your brain isn't there to say, *that's not real, you're fine.* You may try to activate the smart part of your brain and try to convince yourself you are fine. That will work for half a second, but the amygdala, the base lizard part of your brain, has first dibs on your emotions and always gets the last word with OCD.

From your perspective, what does OCD look like through the lens of autism?

There are still many studies that are being done on a medical level which are far beyond my pay grade, but in my experience, being autistic amplifies the obsessiveness of OCD. As I mentioned, hyper-fixation is an autistic trait; it's like a little form of obsession without real fear involved. You're interested in a particular thing, and you find a great deal of joy in it, so you've already established a bit of that obsessive mechanism there in your brain.

For non-autistic people, if they are interested in a particular thing, like books by Brené Brown or a certain kind of coffee, they will want to consume that interest, and when they're done, they're done. But an autistic person will naturally hyper-fixate and can't leave it alone or just shrug it off as if it didn't matter. So when it comes to an autistic person experiencing something like OCD, it is like hyper-fixation on steroids. You can probably imagine just how much an autistic person may want to rationalize, contemplate or control a scary thought. It's almost impossible for them to resist the obsessive cycle because that's often not in their make up on a genetic level.

Why do you think it is so hard to open up and talk about having obsessive compulsive thoughts?

I assume at the root of it for a lot of people there is denial.

You don't want to admit it or acknowledge the thoughts because they are scary, and talking about them makes them feel real. That is crucial, because you are constantly living with that fear. You want to run from it and avoid it as much as humanly possible because it is quite literally your biggest fear in the world. That is why it is stuck in your head in the first place. And in truth, at least from my personal experience, when you acknowledge it at all, even to yourself, you feel like an insane person.

If you have an obsessive thought about something horrendous, like molesting a child, your prefrontal cortex may tell you it's not going to happen, but with OCD the stress signals from your brain are still being sent out and producing extreme anxiety as if that worst possible thing could happen.

It scares you to think of telling someone because you already think you might be crazy. And then you think, if I tell someone *this is my obsessive thought,* they are going to want to lock you up in a mental institution, which can be a common way OCD is misdiagnosed and penalized in an ill-informed society.

For me, I'm sure there were a litany of things that inhibited communication as a kid such as being anxious, feeling like I didn't want to disappoint anyone, or saying something crazy that I couldn't even make sense of myself. As a child I don't think I fully felt open to express myself, even if I did understand what was going on with my thoughts. I was young, and I felt I couldn't express it without a parent either being frustrated, not understanding, or more concerningly wanting to problem-solve.

Ironically, because of my parents' problem-solving nature, I feel like I didn't have the tools to solve my own problems even if I had been able to put my finger on the issue. I didn't know there was a name for what I was experiencing. I thought, like a lot of people with OCD, *Oh I'm just crazy since I just can't stop thinking about it; it's either going to happen or I'm an insane person.*

I think that idea came in part because in the movies, even semi-lighthearted ones, characters who had "obsessive thoughts" were often portrayed as doing the things they thought of so much and enjoying it, like Freddy Krueger or Michael Myers characters from those slasher films. That really seems to be the modern-day representation of intrusive thoughts. So when you actually experience them for yourself and your only frame of reference is sensationalized movie killers who assert, *I just think of murder all the time,* or even the preeminent OCD cliché of a person washing their hands twenty-five times because they are afraid of catching a life-threatening disease, it's pretty hard to be open and honest and tell someone you are having intrusive thoughts.

I didn't know how to validate my feelings about my intrusive thoughts or how to say, *this is how I'm feeling, it's okay just to sit with it for a bit* because I felt fundamentally unwell. It was only after being bottled up for so long, and could not handle it anymore, I told my parents that I was terrified I was going to kill myself. Though I had no desire to do so, the intrusive thoughts kept persisting. When I finally told my mom, I sobbed and felt like the world was collapsing.

I will probably mention this at least a dozen times throughout this book, but as we started to really discover the things that were going on with Isaiah, from Asperger's to anxiety, to Codependency, and then OCD, it initially seemed really hard to grasp. Everything about Isaiah's personality as a young boy was compliant and well-behaved, and in no way did we feel as parents that we were forcing that type of behavior from him; he just seemed to come that way. He was just a really easy-going kid, but as layers began to unfold, we finally began to understand that while his outer way of being was easy-going and compliant, his inner thoughts and emotions were in turmoil.

Even now, as I listen to Isaiah answer these questions with complete truth and honesty, I think back to how things were in his day-to-day life. He talks about an OCD theme called "Just right" OCD and how he used to feel that if he didn't do thirteen hours worth of school work, he was deeply concerned something bad would happen. Of course I had no idea that was how he felt. I remember talking with him at that time about not needing to dwell so much on his homework because he was doing a great job, and even his homeschool teacher spoke with him and said the same. Regardless, he kept doing it. None of us had any idea what the issue really was. When he eventually shared his deep fear of when he went back to in-person class, I was shocked, because not only had his teacher recommended that he skip eighth grade due to his excellent marks, it seemed to me that Isaiah just didn't fail at anything academically, so it never would have dawned on me or any of us for that matter that there was something causing him to feel differently. Thankfully we now know he is autistic, but at the time we didn't know and definitely didn't understand that being autistic left him feeling incapable of communicating what was truly going on.

The fact that now, at twenty-three, Isaiah can fully articulate what he is feeling and thinking in any situation is such a tremendous blessing. This ability would not have taken place if it hadn't been for Isaiah's initial willingness to take steps in understanding his mental health, along with the counselors and psychiatrist who took the time to listen, learn, evaluate and explain things along the way. Additionally, the many individuals who share their personal experiences with being on the spectrum through social media have been a tremendous help in contextualizing and humanizing autism.

All these various professionals, lay people, and resources that we now have, truly show God's fingerprints in Isaiah's life and ours. While we were clueless for so long, God never was, and for that, I am grateful.

You know when I sit and when I rise;
you perceive my thoughts from afar.
You discern my going out and my lying down; you are
familiar with all my ways.

–Psalm 139:2–3

Part II

Going from the initial diagnosis of this thing called Asperger's, which I really knew nothing about, to eventually getting clarification that Asperger's wasn't just its own, isolated thing but actually part of a much broader thing called the Autism Spectrum, felt foreign and just kind of big overall being that it was all so new to me. As foreign as it was and as big as it initially felt, I assumed it would be more or less manageable. Like with most things—especially when it comes to my kids—if there is ever some sort of new variable to what we typically deal with, my goal as Mama is to seek God first then find out as much information as I can in order to guide my babies through all of it, even if they are adult babies.

As I began to learn a bit about the Autism Spectrum, my mama nature wanted to quickly narrow it down and solve it somehow. That's what I assumed would be best to help my son, but the more I tried that familiar approach, the wider the issue seemed to get. I couldn't do my usual attack approach. Instead I had to exercise extreme patience and maintain a flexible mindset that was willing to learn. It didn't take too long for it to become clear to me that I couldn't help my son *through this;* I had to be a student of the spectrum in order to best support my son *in it.* I thought I was doing a fair job of it, but then came OCD.

I thought I knew about OCD before my son was diagnosed with it. Like many people, I believed if you had OCD, then you were a person who wanted everything extremely organized, structured, and lined up. Spices in cupboards would need to be perfectly straight and alphabetized, clothes had to fit just right, and your posture absolutely had to be exceptionally erect. I truly assumed that everything down to your walk had to be just-so for a person with OCD. In other words, I understood Obsessive Compulsive Disorder to be a person who was a bit anal with very obvious ticks and quirks that ultimately revolved around extreme order.

Also like many people, I came to that understanding from the way OCD was portrayed in movies and television. But boy oh boy did the movies and shows I had seen lead me astray.

According to the *National Institute of Mental Health*, Obsessive Compulsive Disorder, or OCD, *"is often a long-lasting disorder in which a person has uncontrollable, reoccurring thoughts (obsessions), and behaviors (compulsions) that he or she feels the urge to repeat over and over."* Many mental health resources confirm that this disorder affects 2.5 million adults or 1.2% of the U.S. population with an average diagnosis age of nineteen years old.

If I'm honest, Asperger's, anxiety, autism and the broad spectrum didn't really scare me. I understood anxiety because I had personally dealt with that in my younger years. While unfamiliar with Asperger's and the spectrum, I was now learning about it, so that felt okay; it felt manageable. But when it came to OCD and how it played out in my son's young life, that terrified me.

I don't know any mom that wouldn't hit a complete inner panic button when her child, whether young or old, says, *"I'm afraid I'm going to kill myself."*

I will never forget that moment. We didn't know about OCD yet, but that night, I walked into my son's room and saw the distressed look on his face. When I asked him what was wrong, he began to sob uncontrollably. Through his tears he finally told me what had been plaguing his mind for so long.

Mom, I'm afraid I'm going to kill myself.

I remember how it felt to hold him in that moment—his tears, his shaking body, the expression of inner turmoil and pain on his face. He was an adult, but he first and foremost was my son, my baby. And as my baby cried and cried, I held him and assured him that we were going to seek help first thing in the morning and that he was going to be alright. As I offered my son comfort, I quietly lifted my own fears to God, asking for the comfort, strength, and wisdom I needed in that moment to help my son with what I completely did not understand. I also prayed that I wasn't wrong and that he really would be alright.

As I was writing the above, I had to stop for a little while because my emotions were getting the better of me. I went to my son's room, walked in, and flopped on his bed. I just needed to cry for a few minutes. Thankfully he was taking a break from his own writing and was able to listen to me explain how I needed to stop writing for a bit because I was reliving the moment a little too vividly.

With tears, I told Isaiah, *I thank God for watching after you and taking care of you.* And true to his quick wit nature, he responded with a humorous, *Who are you telling, sister?*

Fortunately, that frightening breakdown that evening set Isaiah on a trajectory of healing that he didn't even know he needed. Taking that first step of confessing aloud what we later found out were intrusive thoughts—a key symptom of OCD—allowed Isaiah to seek specific counsel and in turn understand for himself what was going on in his mind. After opening up to specialists, he was relieved to discover that he wasn't crazy after all, he just had a disorder that needed to be understood and properly managed.

"I might hit developmental and societal milestones in a different order than my peers, but I am able to accomplish these small victories on my own time."

—Haley Moss, Attorney
Autism Spectrum Award Winner 2019

Within a couple years of your diagnosis of Obsessive Compulsive Disorder, you decided to confront it through a treatment called NOCD. What exactly is NOCD?

NOCD, which stands for *No OCD*, is a program that focuses on compulsion prevention and was originated by Stephen Smith from Chicago, who was frustrated with the lack of treatment resources and support available during his own OCD recovery.

The program was designed to give treatment by OCD-trained, licensed mental health professionals specifically, as contrasted to conventional talk therapy. The whole thing about OCD is that you have one of several irrational, repetitive fears that you try desperately to push away. However, that very action causes the fears to only come back stronger. That's the nature of OCD.

The NOCD program provides a one-on-one counselor that meets with you once or twice a week, and teaches you how to face those fears in incremental forms. Depending how far you are in the program, they help you develop and engage in what are called exposures. The term Exposure Therapy consists of gradually exposing yourself to your fears and helping you habituate and slowly get used to them, even though it feels impossible at first glance.

How did you first learn about this treatment?

I was having one of the hardest episodes I'd had since I

originally got diagnosed with OCD, and I was so frightened by it all. Until that episode, I was too terrified to even look up information or recommendations for help online because I didn't want to admit that it was real. During that episode, I just couldn't take it any more. I reached a point of thinking very clearly to myself, F*** this, and I took the plunge to begin looking for help. I eventually came across a series of YouTube videos by an OCD Specialist named Nathan Peterson, whose channel was dedicated to talking about OCD, and I found it very helpful. I was amazed and encouraged by the fact that I was able to even look up videos about OCD and that it didn't crumble my entire world. Better yet, it didn't give me terrible anxiety to get through the videos. From there, things sort of snowballed from me watching his videos to me looking up an OCD activity workbook to see what I could do to get help. It was through that series that I first learned about exposures. I was able to get a more structured look at OCD and exposures through a workbook that I found on Amazon titled, *The Complete OCD Workbook* by Scott Granet. I could tell it was something that would help me stay more organized and accountable. I needed this type of format because I knew if I only worked on getting better when I felt like it or was in the mood to do an exposure, it wouldn't happen, because the reality is you are never in the mood to interact with your deepest fears.

The nature of an exposure is to make you uncomfortable and to build up your tolerance for it. That's why when one of my previous therapists recommended a book, not a workbook but one to read about OCD, of course I didn't want to read it at the time. I didn't want to engage with anything having to do with OCD. I was a lot more open to working through a workbook written by a clinician who personally understood how frightening exposures were and wrote the book for people like me, who were engaging with OCD for the first time.

It felt that Granet wrote it specifically for readers with OCD to simply understand and finally be willing to jump into the deep end of the pool, so to speak, but still have some degree of their wits about them. For many people like myself, when you first learn you have OCD, you know as much about it as the average person, which is very little. Knowing so little is a tremendous hindrance because you *have* it and it's highly debilitating.

That's how I basically began learning about exposure and response prevention (ERP), the official term of OCD exposure therapy. I didn't have any referral. I just began searching for different OCD treatments and online programs. I finally found NOCD and was happy to realize the treatment might actually be covered by my insurance. I was able to talk with an insurance representative pretty quickly who was very nice, and she explained to me that because OCD is broadly recognized in medical and psychiatric associations as a legitimate disorder that requires treatment, my insurance would indeed cover NOCD.

Can you describe an OCD episode you experienced for better understanding for those who don't know?

The worst episode I had that finally led me to research information about OCD online revolved around my recurrent fear of me killing myself. The thoughts would come intensely, then go away, then reoccur. That was the same fear I had when

I was nineteen and initially got diagnosed with OCD. I was terrified that I was going to impulsively kill myself by driving my car off the freeway. Anytime I drove on the freeway I was constantly thinking, *What if I just drive off?* It felt as if it *was* happening because my amygdala (lizard brain) doesn't respond to rationality or frontal cortex, and thus it sends out genuine distress signals. It felt like the end of the world with no amount of reasoning or rationale fixing available. In addition to the fear of running off the road as a way of killing myself, there were other scenarios generated by the same fear.

I could see a pair of scissors and think, *What if I stab myself in the neck with them?* I could see a pencil and think the same but with added details such as, *What if I stab myself with a pencil in the neck and choke on splinters and die?* I was like a very morbid version of the TV show MacGyver, given how innovative I was in imagining all the ways I could fulfill my greatest fear. The more I tried to resist the fearful thoughts, the harder it got. I compared it to Chinese finger traps where you put your fingers in the bamboo tube, and the more you try to pull them out, the more the tube constricts.

The intrusive thoughts would come, and I would keep trying to pull away in the most logical ways I could think of. I would try to distract myself or tell myself that everything was fine; but the brain is exceptionally headstrong when it thinks it's saving you from danger. When it comes to chemicals in your brain relating to fear, the brain can produce them a lot quicker than it produces rational thought, particularly when experiencing a neurological feature such as OCD.

Being that you were already seeing a therapist who was familiar with Asperger's, autism and OCD, why did you choose NOCD for treatment instead of just working through it with the therapist you were seeing?

I needed a very specific fix. When you have OCD it feels like the end of the world, and you need someone who understands that fact *very* clearly and very specifically. It's not something where you want any type of meditative advice, it feels extremely urgent and important to get the right kind of help. The therapist I was already seeing was familiar with OCD but not on a personal level. A big part of what helped with my healing experience was that my NOCD counselor had OCD, so he could relate to how terrifying it all felt since he was in the same boat.

Even though my counselor prior to the NOCD program was entirely right when she said, "Have you considered just allowing the thought?" I couldn't take a suggestion so broad; my brain needed to break down the pieces of *how* I could possibly allow that thought. What type of thoughts should I allow? Do you start with baby steps? I needed it broken down because I didn't know how to step at all. She was entirely correct in what she said, but wasn't able to empathize, only sympathize. And that makes a huge difference especially when it's such a personal form of grief where you feel as if you were going crazy, which seems to be the most common feeling I've seen among people with OCD.

Can you describe the NOCD steps that you personally went through?

NOCD uses Exposure Response Prevention (ERP) as their main form of treatment, and the general rule of thumb for ERP is that you are exposed to a fear, and you work to prevent your usual response of trying to block that fear, fix your feelings, or reassure yourself.

To my understanding, ERP is provided roughly the same way across all OCD treatment programs worth their salt. The way ERP was approached through NOCD was by having me build a *hierarchy* or write down every single thing I was afraid could happen. For example, *What if I kill my kid? What if I keep feeling the urge to kill my kid? Oh my god, I am a terrible person. I can't, this is just terrible. I keep having this violent thought of killing my kid.* If you have a specific fear like that, then by building a hierarchy and writing every single thing down, you can for one, identify it, and then you identify all the triggers, meaning all the things that make you think about killing your kid or in my case, killing myself.

Doing this helped to realize that I had specific triggers, otherwise the entire world seemed like an overwhelming trigger. When I began to identify triggers, I realized any type of weapon, sharp objects, pen, etc., were some of mine. Ugh, I could tell you a litany of things that I had thought of killing myself with because that's how my OCD brain goes. It's imagining a thousand paths to the same dreaded destination.

When you are writing your list, you're looking for every single trigger you can think of. It could be something that happens in a social interaction or something you see in a movie where someone does the thing you fear, or even a song with lyrics that touch upon what's making you unhappy. Whatever it is that affects you personally *is* the trigger. Another for me was any TV show or movie that involved suicide.

That's actually what happened with the popular Netflix show, *You*. I watched it once and saw that one episode included a suicide warning. Unsurprisingly, I avoided it like the plague for months, but when I started doing exposures I forced myself to try again. I ended up loving the show. I don't even remember if there was a full suicide scene or not, but I was so proud of the fact that I was willing to step closer to my fear.

So yes, you start by writing down all of your fears, every single one that you think of, every single thing that has ever scared you. That's it. You don't have to face them. You don't have to do anything crazy yet, because acknowledging them alone can be plenty frightening. Just write them down.

From there you assign a number value of least scary to most scary to each item on your list. Your scale could be one through ten or one through one hundred, whatever is most comfortable. Some people prefer numbering one to one hundred because it really gets you to specifically express how severe a fear is, while a small scale of on to ten can seem benign.

If your scale is one to one hundred, then you rank each trigger, with one being a little scary and one hundred being Mount Kilimanjaro, a kind of scary that you could never imagine facing. That's what I did, and it is roughly what people do in general with NOCD. You really want to take your time. It is not something you have to do in ten minutes. Take a day or take a week. Consider every fear you have, then just write it out, along with every trigger that sparks the fear.

Once you are done writing your list and ranking your fears, a specialist takes your list and organizes a hierarchy. They put the list in order of easiest to scariest, then help you willfully engage with a low grade trigger. It's not fun, but it's the most effective treatment I've ever experienced.

There's no limit to the number of things you have on your list, or the ranking. It's just a spectrum. I've had more than one fear on my list that was neck in neck, with another in terms of severity. One fear might rank at a seventy-four and the other a seventy-five but it really doesn't matter. Just be as honest as you can.

At that point, your specialist will talk to you through specifically what an exposure will look like for the various items on your list.

To give one example: Harm OCD is when you specifically have a fear that you will harm yourself or someone else. I was so spooked by even the concept of self harm. I began by just writing down the word *suicide*. It's a modest but potent confrontation with this element of fear that has, up till now, dictated the sufferer's life. Still, it scares you; but that's fine, it's supposed to. Your goal is to take one step at a time, despite the fear.

Each little step teaches your brain to kind of become a brute and to work *through* the unpleasant feelings. Since we can't rationalize our way out of fears for good, people with OCD have to make concerted efforts to desensitize their brains to triggers.

That is the abnormality of the OCD brain. Since you can't go through reason, you have to go through brute strength. And through brute mental strength you'll do the same scary thing over and over and over again until your brain slowly understands, *Oh I don't need to keep sending out the same chemicals over this.* When my brain continually sent out cortisol, a stress hormone, over and over because I was writing the word suicide, and I didn't try do anything to fight away the fear, it eventually stopped becoming a fight. In other words you're not trying to pull your fingers out of Chinese finger traps anymore—you are just relaxing until they slip off.

I have often heard it recommended that people should smile while they're doing things they dislike because smiling produces happier hormones, and slowly but steadily builds a positive association with the things you dislike. When I say this is a concerted effort, I mean it is all hands on deck to change your neurological behavior.

Similarly with NOCD, once you finish doing an exposure counselors recommend you do something enjoyable to make you remember the experience as a good thing. Personally, I would play a video game afterwards or listen to a song I really liked to make sure I had a positive association with the very trying task, otherwise I wouldn't want to go through it again.

As you have described the beginning steps of the NOCD program, would you say anyone struggling with OCD can do these steps on their own or should they have a NOCD specialist walk them through?

In my opinion, you should definitely have a specialist walk you through the steps because it's so easy to not recognize how or when you're doing a compulsion. For example you may have a thought about killing yourself and not recognize that you also tend to tell yourself, *Just kidding,* to push away the stress. There are so many things we don't realize are compulsions that a counselor or specialist who is trained to see from an impartial point of view can see, whereas those of us struggling with OCD are always going to have perceptions filtered by our own fear.

Having a specialist guide you through is extremely helpful. You don't need one forever, and that's by design, because they help you develop tools to be much more self-aware and independent. This understanding is crucial so you don't develop some bad habits that could prevent the ERP from being successful.

It has been some time since you initially worked through the NOCD program. Do you still find yourself regularly using the same tools?

I would say once you get so used to it, it goes beyond just specific tools and instead becomes a general mindset of trying to go closer toward the things that make you uncomfortable. Not because you like it but because it gives you a head start, at least that is how I try to think of it. It puts you in control of the narrative. Not that you can control your feelings, but you can majorly influence whether or not it becomes debilitating because you keep avoiding the problem, or if it becomes much more doable because you deal with it in the short term. So yes, I have definitely used it on random occasions when I find something comes up, but it really is a mindset now, and it is a lot easier to not only recognize triggers but to move closer to them. That is what I primarily focus on because there was such a long period of time where I might recognize a trigger, but wouldn't do anything about it except run away from it.

A perfect example of this would be when I experienced one form of OCD called *Disgust OCD*. Disgust OCD is where you suffer intrusive thoughts of repulsive images or ideas. Before NOCD, if exposed to something disgusting it would have triggered endless thoughts like, *What if I keep thinking of this and I'm never able to do anything else? What if I'm never happy again because I'm only ever thinking about this gross thing?* It was predictably uncomfortable, so I sought to avoid it by distracting myself.

Now, even if I have a brief moment of thinking about something disgusting, I recognize that I don't want to think about it, but I also understand that I might. And so I'll try and give myself at least a moment to walk closer toward it, and specifically try to think about that gross thing that *seems* unbearable. Fortunately it has not become a consistent theme, only something that might come up every few weeks if that, but now I'm more likely to let a thought come and go without concern. I don't want to run away from it or have it become this lingering boogeyman, so I walk closer towards it.

You have mentioned how during an OCD episode, there is not a natural capability of recognizing that something is not actually a threat. With that in mind, would you say there is a greater level of importance for someone with OCD to confront fears and even sit with their fears a bit versus someone who has fears unrelated to OCD?

Absolutely. It is so important to confront and sit with your fears for a bit, and yes, it's terrifying. You feel terrible, and worse yet, you are the one putting yourself in the situation. Still, doing so without trying to *fix* the fear allows you to work through it little by little. This is why it's important to start small, because initially, even the smallest fear can feel like the end times.

> *Whenever you practiced exposures, you were literally feeling what you needed to feel which was very uncomfortable, and it seemed like it wasn't something I could help you with. Was it important for you that I didn't do the typical mom thing and try to take the uncomfortable feelings away and fix it?*

It was extremely important. You not trying to step in and fix it made the difference between me *getting over* it and going *through* it. A willingness on my part to go through it was pleasing in the sense that I was ready to try, but it was also so difficult, especially doing it for the first time. Fortunately, it does get slightly easier just about every time after that.

Part of what's maddening is that it feels like you're never going to get through. That's the nature of fear; when you're afraid of something, you're not thinking of long-term benefits, you are feeling in the present moment that you are doing something wrong that's putting you in danger.

For me, starting small meant writing the word *suicide* five times, and then ten times, then fifteen. Many times the goal for any exposure is to keep doing it for at least ten minutes. Your stress level is probably going to be pretty high if you're doing an exposure for the first time. You might be at a seventy percent feeling of fear and anxiety and not want to keep going, but out of spite for the difficulties of OCD, you don't stop.

Next time you write the word you might be at seventy percent feeling of fear and anxiety again, but after a few minutes it goes down to sixty-five percent. You are still feeling a lot of fear, but that is improvement.

The goal with exposures is to wait until your anxiety calms down by about half of where you started at. So if you start at seventy percent feeling anxiety while doing the exposure and wait to get down to about thirty-five percent, that's fine. You don't have to get rid of all of your anxiety, *you are just trying to manage it.* If you can get it down to a ten to fifteen percent, that's awesome, but getting it down by half of whatever you usually experience is generally considered a success. To compare coming down from one hundred percent anxiety rate when you're thinking, *This is it, I'm about to die, this is the end of my life, the end of everything I love,* down to fifty percent where you think, *I don't like this, this is scary,* but you still have of your wits about you; that's a huge difference. That difference will begin to show in your day-to-day life.

During my first session I started writing *suicide* on paper with seventy percent fear and eventually was able to get down to thirty-five. In session two, again I started at seventy but came down thirty percent. Session three I went from sixty down to thirty. By the fourth session I went from fifty percent down to twenty percent.

As you work through the exposure, you may feel capable of picking a fear to address that is lower down on your list. Instead of picking something that you ranked as a twenty out of one hundred, you might be challenged by your counselor to try something you ranked as thirty out of a one hundred. As daunting as it feels, this is progress.

I was fortunate enough to be very open to the experience. When I talked to my counselor, he joked about how "I was the only person who had ever taken notes during a session." Honestly, I took notes because I was so sick of OCD. It was just the worst thing I'd ever experienced, worse than my relationship breakup, mourning, and physical pain combined. I was really quite assiduous in trying to combat OCD by getting to the point of saying, *I am scared, but let's try, because I'm tired of being scared.* I felt I had nothing to lose.

My mind was constantly spread thin. Not even just busy but incapable of focusing, incapable of *enjoying* things, because every chemical in my brain was dedicated to being afraid. Trying to navigate around that fear as if I had control over it was impossible, so it was a big benefit to finally reach a point of being so sick of it all that I was willing to try.

Part of your NOCD treatment included an online support group, and in that group there were many older people who were dealing with their OCD for the first time. Is it beneficial to seek help for OCD if you are much older, or is it almost too late?

It's never too late as long as you're willing. I mean really, do you want to be better than miserable? That's the question for someone struggling with OCD no matter what age.

That particular NOCD online support group was about mental compulsions, and most of the people in that particular group were in their fifties and sixties and almost all of them were just getting help for the first time in their lives. This type of support is something that is just now becoming available. I was lucky to have *any* help available online, but even then, it wasn't like the internet was brimming with resources. There was *one* YouTube channel that I used often and *one* online service of NOCD, and that was in the year 2021. The iPhone had been invented, and we've been to the moon, yet we still struggle to provide even mediocre service for people with debilitating disorders like OCD. Having any kind of resource was a big thing for me in my early twenties, let alone for the people in my support group who were in their fifties and sixties.

Forty years ago if someone said they had intrusive thoughts of killing themself or thought of getting AIDS from not washing their hands enough, the best that might happen if they mustered the courage to plead for help, was that loved ones and medical institutions could largely dismiss and stigmatize the sufferer. It's understandable, even now, because people just don't have an interest in the reality of this disorder. Unfortunately, sufferers will go decades of just thinking, *Well I guess this is my life*—and then get worse because they keep training themselves in new ways to avoid their fears.

Does having continual intrusive thoughts mean you will act upon them when you have OCD?

No. An intrusive thought like, *I'm afraid I'm going to hurt somebody,* does not make the person with OCD more inclined to actually hurt someone. But even having those horrid thoughts is why people with OCD often judge themselves so harshly.

There's a whole chapter in *The Complete OCD Workbook* by Scott Granet on cognitive distortions; things that steadily warp your perception of yourself, and one of them is thought-action fusion, which is thinking about something that leads you to treat yourself as if you have done it. For someone with OCD, they might think about punching someone in the face and then feel extremely guilty as if they did it. You completely forget that there's a stark difference between *thinking* about punching someone and actually causing harm by doing it.

Another is emotional reasoning, which means the sufferer has a conscious or unconscious belief that if it *feels* like I'm gonna do it, it must mean I'm gonna do it. *I feel it in my gut* is often the excuse people use as to why they do a compulsion like washing their hands for an hour. It's that they feel anxiety in their gut, so they have to keep themselves safe. Problem being, OCD hijacks your "gut feeling" to be hyperactive.

That's the whole thing with OCD, all these chemicals in the brain are making them constantly think; *I'm gonna do it in a split second. I'm about to do this thing right now,* and they literally never do.

On the other hand, someone with frequent visceral thoughts of violence who does not have OCD or any other pertinent anxiety disorder will never *worry* about if they are going to do something harmful—they just do it. When's the last time you met a truly crazy person, who said *I wonder if I'm crazy?* People like Ted Bundy, or Ted Kaczynski never said, *I wonder if I will hurt someone?* They don't worry about it, because the notion of harm is fine with them, contrary to those with OCD.

It's a specific fear, and you do compulsions to push away the fear, but it keeps coming back. That's what makes it a compulsive *disorder.* If you're afraid that you're going to denounce God, and I don't mean just a crisis–of–faith moment, because a crisis of faith is normal, but if you're chronically afraid you're gonna denounce God but have no actual desire to, and you're thinking, *What if I denounce God? What if I prefer the devil? What if I go to hell?* and so on, one thing you might do to reassure yourself is to say certain prayers over and over to try and feel godly. It's a very routine thing, it's very easy to become ritualistic beyond just a religious practice but to *fix* something in order to feel better. You're not doing it out of a genuine place, you're doing it until it feels *just right* so you don't have that fear anymore. You're doing it not to be a good person, but to push away the intrusive thoughts and feelings.

Sometimes, you see people with OCD who are very peaceful people and value life but have terrible fears of harming someone else, and the thought immediately snowballs into, *I shouldn't think about that*, but then they naturally can't stop the thought and start pushing it away, even though it's something they wouldn't do to begin with. Their thought is *born* out of fear, and it snowballs into this huge mountain of fear when it's avoided. They keep trying to avoid it so much that this extremely peaceful person who would never want to do it has this ego-dystonic experience where they are terrified that they are split seconds away from harming someone. Unmanaged, OCD can truly torment a person's thoughts, but that's a world away from acting on their tormented thoughts.

At any point did you feel NOCD wasn't going to help you, or did you feel it would help right from the start?

I wish I could have had that much of a thought process. When you're scared out of your mind, you don't think clearly. You're in a constant state of anxiety and all of the fear and anxiety agitation which inhibits complex thinking. So I wasn't in a place to think, *Oh this is gonna be helpful for XYZ reasons.* This was me just taking steps, very small steps, and saying, *I really hope this works because I don't like OCD.* I was just hoping it got better, because my brain was carrying too much weight. Just existing as a person is a lot at times for anyone, but having the massive anxiety of OCD and dealing with it all as an autistic person was really a lot. Then adding the idea of exposure therapy, not knowing if it would work, but realizing I'm going to have to face these fears and be closer to them as part of the process made me all the more anxious. So yeah. I had no idea, I was just hoping.

What was the turning point while doing the NOCD program that you realized it would actually help?

As much as it would be nice and simple to think that at some point everything just clicks, and you don't have to be afraid, it doesn't work like that. You constantly have little moments during an exposure of finding it scary and still feeling terrified to do the next one. After so many moments of terror while practicing exposures, I was finally able to look back and have some sense of getting somewhere. Slowly, that built up the realization that I was able to look at things that formerly triggered me with a newfound indifference. However, there was never a specific turning point where I realized, *Oh I'm getting the hang of this, this is definitely going to work.* I really didn't know that it was going to be helpful. I guess like anything in life, hindsight is twenty-twenty. You just take the steps and keep going down the road until you are able to get a little bit of distance and perspective to look back and see some sort of progress.

It's the benefit of holding yourself accountable, it's not just so that you do something in the first place but that you recognize that you have accomplished it afterward. I think that was eventually a big part of me taking notes, because I knew it would be a record for later, of things I'd successfully done. I would take pictures of the assignments my counselor gave me each week and favorite them on my phone so they were always very accessible. I would see them months later for whatever reason and think, *Wow, I just don't even care about that particular thing like I once did. It's not triggering or even relevant anymore.*

Tell me about the trigger reminders you purposely put on your phone?

I put reminders on my phone for months. They were designed to be exposures. Anything that would scare me, concern me or make me feel unhappy. I did this because I realized my obsessive concern went from, *What if I impulsively kill myself?* to *What if I want to kill myself?* And then eventually to, *What if I am just fundamentally unhappy forever?* So I put reminders in my phone that would come up hourly, designed to promote that fear. I wouldn't get a warning ahead of time, the reminder would just pop up. One reminder would say, "suicide." An hour or so later a reminder would pop up that said, "you might never be happy." Then another reminder would pop up with, "you might never find love, that's a possibility."

It wasn't even about finding a way to accept the fearful reminders, because people with OCD very often try to think through things and find some sort of mental way around what they're afraid of or rationalize it. Really I just had to let sleeping dogs lie. If the reminder said "suicide," I was eventually able just look at it and think, *Oh suicide.* If the reminder said, "kill yourself," I would look at it and think, *I just have to keep going through my day.* I don't get to fix it, or try to delete it, or tell myself, "just kidding." I wasn't going to do any of that. I just needed to see it and then let it go.

I know you touched upon this already, and it's such a natural instinct for moms to want to protect their children from anything unpleasant, but that really doesn't seem to work with OCD does it?

Exactly. Following maternal impulses is helpful if your kid is going to get hit by a car, and you swoop in to save them, but there is also a time for letting someone feel their own feelings, like when the kid cries at the realization that they almost got hit by a car. At that moment, it doesn't benefit them for you to say something like, *You are going to be okay, I promise it will never happen again,* just so their scared feelings will go away. They have to be allowed to feel their feelings without an instant fix or solution. Of course if they have irrational anxiety about it in the future, you might say, *I'm so sorry you feel that way. I'm here for you. I can't take your feelings for you, but I support you.* In that way, you are allowing the child to feel their scary feelings while knowing they are still supported. That's exactly the kind of support I needed when it came to OCD and autism.

I've often heard counselors use the term, "Let's reframe that" in regards to turning a negative thought into a positive one. Based on what you have been sharing, reframing a negative thought is not always the best thing for someone dealing with OCD, is that correct?

As frustrating as it was, I had to learn that the healthiest perspective I could have would be to take problems for what they were—nothing more or less. If you say, *I stepped on someone's toe, and that means I want to hurt them,* and then you try to reframe it as, *I only barely stepped on their toes, so I'm really a good person,* you are just going from beating yourself up to reassuring yourself, which only continues the OCD cycle. A middle ground of accepting objective realities is crucial.

If you're reframing something you're not obsessed about but maybe just a touch anxious over, that's fine, be positive, that's genuinely great. But if it's an obsessive thought that you are trying to comfort yourself about by running from the initial thought, that's not really going to help. It's you avoiding your problem.

For me, one benefit to being autistic was the hyper-fixation of wanting to get better. It's a rare benefit, but it really made me want to work hard on it.

When you are hyper-fixated on a task that you're trying to achieve, there can be this sense of, *I'm dying to achieve this so either help me or get out of my way.* When I reached the point of really wanting help with OCD, that was just how it had to be for me, especially because I was so insecure. I had to assert that feeling of, *I'm just going to do this, and if someone doesn't understand, it sucks for them, but they can just get out of my way.* It wasn't even out of contempt that I had this mindset, it was just out of a legitimate concern and desire for well-being within myself.

Would you recommend NOCD to others who have OCD, and is there a specific resource to point them too?

Because I had such personal success with NOCD, I would

highly recommend it. I would also suggest checking with your insurance to see if they cover NOCD treatment which they very well might. But even if they didn't, it's worth it. Before I discovered the NOCD program, I was able to purchase *The Complete OCD Workbook* by Scott Granet through Amazon. That was actually the first thing I had *in my hands* that helped me put pen to paper and really work on OCD in order to try and understand it. That was me really going forward and committing to exposures initially for the first time. When it comes down to it, I believe if anyone with OCD wants to get better, they absolutely can.

There is a small chunk of books, resources, and videos such as the ones I watched on YouTube by Nathan Peterson, LCSW. I watched a lot of his videos, and none of them were reassuring, which was very frustrating as a person who desperately wanted reassurance. But they were extremely informative and helped me understand that I had to work *through* what I was experiencing, not just be reassured.

If money is an issue, I would have to say that one of the most effective things I believe you can do based on my own experience is to make a habit of going a little closer to the things you are afraid of. I highly recommend the guidelines of a book, because the notion of getting closer to things you are afraid of in life in general is very provoking, so doing it with a certain amount of structure can make it feel like you have railing supporting you, but either way, you absolutely can do it.

One of the ways I began to understand the difference between how someone with OCD might think about something versus someone without OCD, was when Isaiah and I were talking about a large cutting knife we have at home.

When my children were little, I would usually make dinner, put all the dirty dishes in the sink, then wash them after we ate. There was usually at least one large cutting knife used for preparing the meal in the sink amongst all the dirty dishes. With little busy-body children around, I got into the safety habit of washing the knife, drying it and putting it away first before tackling the rest of the dishes, so none of us, particularly the children, would bump into the counter, knock over the knife and accidentally cut ourself. This is a pretty rational thought for any parent of little children, but even when all my kids grew up, I didn't change the habit. To this day, if I use a sharp knife to prepare a meal, I still quickly wash, dry, and put it away. Not because I fear the knife, but just for that safety.

When Isaiah started working through NOCD and was finally able to express the intrusive thoughts he was having about the fear of killing himself and how knives were a trigger, one of the things he said he needed from me was to *not* put away the knife. This obviously went against every safety code I had ever practiced as a mom, but this is what he was asking.

It was hard for me to leave a knife out in general, but more so because of his particular intrusive thoughts. Nevertheless, the request made something click for me in regard to understanding the difference between my thoughts about a knife out and Isaiah's. So I did as he requested.

If ever I had considered slacking off when it came to talking to God and presenting Him with my heartfelt prayers, let me tell you that first time, purposely leaving a sharp cutting knife out on the counter so my son could work through his harm OCD exposure squashed the idea of slacking off in my talks with God from ever happening for the rest of my life.

Hearing Isaiah tell me his actual thoughts, *What if I grab a knife and slit my throat? What if I drive right off the road and kill myself?* was not what I wanted to hear. If there were ever moments in life that I would want to be in denial, that would have been the moment, but it was Isaiah's truth. So I listened, and I didn't go into denial. I chose to pray first, then stay open and keep learning about OCD and how autism impacts the disorder.

I know the younger generation today takes a lot of heat for their crazy ways, and yes, they sure do have some crazy ways, but nevertheless, one thing I think they might have figured out a bit better than the older generation who were raised with more of a, *Suck it up and don't talk about it* mentality, is to be open, to learn, to understand, and to express in order to grow.

Once Isaiah understood his initial diagnosis of being on the spectrum and what looking through the lens of autism meant in all areas of his life, including OCD, he became a willing student who was open, ready to learn and understand his mental health. In turn, he was able to help me get as comfortable as I could be with all the uncomfortable things he needed to walk through.

A Word from Nathan Peterson

In the process of writing this book, I decided to reach out to Nathan Person, LCSW via email and see if he would mind sharing a brief word on the importances of addressing OCD. I didn't know how likely it was that I would actually connect with him as I was certain he was a pretty busy man. Turns out he was indeed very busy and was in the midst of traveling, yet he still took the time to respond with some powerful words of wisdom about addressing OCD.

"If we don't understand how OCD functions, we won't know how to fight it. Just like most things in life. Taking time to understand the error messages, triggers, compulsions, and interferences in life are important. Many waste their time trying to understand the "content." Meaning, why am I worried about this? Will I really do this thing? Is it because of my childhood? etc. The fear the individual has doesn't matter. What matters is their brain is taking a thought that most people have and flagging it as dangerous.

"It's our job to teach these error messages that they aren't dangerous, and that is through exposure and response prevention. We do this little by little. We are facing fears. I'll use an example that may be outside of the OCD realm and that many can relate to.

"If I'm afraid of spiders, I'm not going to jump into a tank full of spiders. I'm going to think about the spider

until it's boring. Look at a picture of one. Read stories about them. Watch videos of them. Play with fake spiders. Be close to one and maybe get to the point of touching it. I may be doing this over weeks. My brain is throwing out danger messages, and I'm acting as if they don't matter, thus teaching the brain that it doesn't need to keep sending them.

"If I went straight to the tank of spiders, my brain may not learn much. If I did it little by little, my brain is learning overtime that the only value it has is what we give it.

Treatment takes time. It's a muscle that needs to be strengthened and used often. It needs to, and can be, mastered."

"The Lord walks beside me—He renews my strength. He guides me along right paths, bringing honor to his name. Even when I walk through the darkest valley, I will not be afraid, for you are close beside me."

–Psalm 23:3–4

Part III

Discovering a Sense of Self

In 2019 when my son transferred as a junior to a university four hundred miles away, I knew I would miss him terribly, but I was also excited for him because I genuinely believed he would have the time of his life. It had been about a year since we learned he was autistic, and we were still in the midst of discovering what exactly that meant, but we were not too concerned as he had a counselor in place to support him. He had such a strong desire to get his film degree from this particular school, so we felt confident it was the right choice for him. He was nineteen years old, and I assumed his first taste of freedom on a seemingly safe campus would bring him great joy. I had pictured him busting out of his quiet reserved way and making life-long friends on the very first day of school. I assumed he would settle in quickly and was eager to buy him all those little items college kids typically get from their parents when they head to their dorms for the first time. To be honest, my biggest worry was that my son might actually have such a great time right from the start that he wouldn't end up needing his mama quiet so much any more. As all moms who send their child off to college for the first time know, that's a rough feeling to go through, but I also knew it was an important step for his life, his growth, and his personal self-discovery.

Isaiah's uncle was the one to drop him off at his dorm on his first day on campus while my husband and I went to work and tried to be brave. His proud uncle texted me a picture that he took of Isaiah using his keycard to unlock his door for the very first time. When I opened the text and saw the picture, a part of me wanted to cry, but a bigger part wanted to puff my chest out a bit with a good dose of mama pride as I thought, *Today my son's new journey begins.* No more than ten minutes later, that thought turned into a massive understatement.

Isaiah had secured a position with the college newspaper which was well regarded on and off campus. Being that he loved writing and was majoring in film, he was eager to be a part of the college newspaper as well. We naturally assumed he would be writing articles about new students, dorm-life, sports, and all sorts of campus activities.

The plan that first day was that he would settle into his dorm, then make his way over to the newsroom later in the afternoon. However, about ten minutes into being on campus and arriving at his dorm, he received a 911 sort of text from the newspaper editor stating that a staff member had been murdered on campus approximately one hour earlier, and the police were searching for the suspect. The editor asked my son to drop everything and immediately head to the office. Rushing at breakneck speed to the newsroom turned out to be Isaiah's intro to college life.

Needless to say, for months, this tragedy dominated most of what my son wrote about, thought about, and researched for the newspaper. From this startling situation, we learned something very significant about Isaiah's autistic nature. He can easily go down a rabbit hole, so to speak, and become extremely engrossed and all-consumed when it comes to issues of injustice. Obviously the murder of a faculty member in the parking lot near the newsroom was the ultimate injustice, which made Isaiah's desire for research go beyond the newspaper's needs. It seemed to me on the outside looking in, gathering the information was somehow personal for Isaiah, especially once the police caught the suspect who was also a fellow faculty member.

Maybe it sounds heroic in some way that my son wanted to find out all he could to help beyond just a newspaper story, but from a concerned parent's point of view, it didn't feel heroic. At a certain point, it felt concerning. Perhaps more so, because our son was autistic and had yet to fully learn how this and other aspects of the spectrum could affect him, let alone just being a young person who was completely unaware of his sense of self at that point.

As my son went down the rabbit hole of research, the stress caused him to be who he is in regards to his hyper-fixation, but not necessarily understood, at least not by those he worked with, and that began to cause problems for him. As for me, his mom, my overwhelming concern was, *How do I get my son out of this rabbit hole? How do I get others to understand him and to understand his very well-meaning ways?*

Turns out I didn't really need to find the answer to those questions as COVID-19 shut everything down and brought my son back home months later. While he did gain a significant measure of independence being away from us for seven months, the tragedy of murder, his rabbit hole response, and a lack of overall connection with others and himself took a toll.

In hindsight, my son was a fish out of water in every way on that campus. It was supposed to be this great, growing experience. Instead it brought about a great deal of stress. I suppose the one positive take away was the stress brought out signs and symptoms that for us as his parents we had never really noticed before. Isaiah has often referred to these signs and symptoms as *little tiny Easter eggs or little bread crumbs for knowing that you are autistic.* And that was exactly what it was like for us. We finally started recognizing the breadcrumbs of his different way of doing things. We no longer had to be *told* he was on the spectrum by doctors, because we were able to see things more clearly for ourselves.

As with most college students around the world at that time, Isaiah came home and completed his college education online. His on-campus college experience was nothing like any of us had hoped or imagined it would be. In fact, it was one extremely challenging period of time that ended up being a springboard into an even more challenging period, as Isaiah began experiencing his OCD symptoms more severely and in a way that he could no longer ignore.

Through it all, the challenges did lead Isaiah to begin discovering his true sense of self. Albeit, in a way that was much harder than anticipated but by God's grace, so very worth it.

"Everyone has a mountain to climb and autism has not been my mountain, it has been my opportunity for victory."

–Rachel Barcellona

Talking with Isaiah

What was your sense of self like before getting diagnosed, and did the diagnosis set you on a path for wanting to gain a sense of self?

I think to a certain degree, getting a diagnosis was a jump starter for me wanting to gain a sense of self. Recently I was watching an analysis of different TV Pilots, since I am now writing one. In it, they discussed dormant characters, such as in the show *Breaking Bad.* In the first episode, the main character, Walter White, is passive and living his life on autopilot, but when he gets diagnosed with cancer it changes his identity and forces him to live purposely. He finds identity in negative choices, which makes for a good show, but for me, getting a diagnosis of autism had a similar, but more positive, effect. Having autism was something where I couldn't just ask someone else to direct me on. I didn't know anyone autistic, and there wasn't really a rule book that could tell me how to be autistic. It was so integral to having a sense of self in general. Having no one else to lead me through being autistic forced me to live purposely and think of what *I* wanted, what *I* preferred, versus being directed by someone else or feeling obligated. Having to take up that responsibility of *Oh yeah, I'm feeling my feelings, and this is what they might stem from,* is something that led to a lot of individuality.

As your mom, at times I have wondered, if I had known earlier that you were autistic and perhaps knew

*other parents with autistic children, could I have led you in some
way that would have made things a bit easier for you?*

I've thought about that, how it could have been different
in childhood if research in general had been more progressive.
If schools had been more familiar with the range of behaviors
for students on the autism spectrum. The school I went to
didn't have any aides for kids on the spectrum. There were
no individual students with aides in the regular classroom,
you just had one class with Special Needs kids, and you never
knew what went on there. They just seemed to vaguely learn
skills and were very much separated from other students.
You saw them here and there like it was a special event. To
be honest, there always seemed to be an insinuation that
they were stupid. I never received any specialized learning
mechanisms, opportunities, or incentives like the kids I work
with now, who use token boards to stay on task, and give
them something to work toward. I didn't have any goal or
initiative other than gaining a teacher's approval or feeling
like I was good enough by doing the right things, which
ultimately proved healthy.

I didn't have any sense of personal achievement, which is
so needed, especially being autistic. If I had been structurally
supported by a fundamentally more sound school system, that
could have massively changed how I was educated and turned
out. Not only intellectually, but it could have really helped
with developing emotional skills and setting a foundation
for that at a young age, whereas just now, I'm having to learn
how to process my feelings as an adult on the spectrum.

There is an expression, "Monday Morning Quarterbacking,"
referring to how most football games take place on Sunday

night, and come Monday morning, quarterbacks rewatch their game with new found clarity and an insatiable desire to go back in time and fix their mistakes. You can do the same with parenting, with school, and so on. Looking back, you realize what you could have done differently because you now know how everything went, and you don't have the same emotional issues you had at that time. You don't experience the same uncertainty, the same coworkers, the same teachers, or the same friends, so you know how to navigate it. You know how everything turns out. That is why I believe Monday Morning Quarterbacking is so natural to do. We all wonder, fight ourselves, wondering, *What if I had done something different in the past?* I imagine especially as a parent, Monday Morning Quarterbacking would come naturally.

Based on your previous experience as a student and your present experience as a substitute in the school district, do you think teachers have a better understanding about Special Needs and are better able to recognize those students who are on the spectrum but may not show obvious symptoms?

If educators had been trained to know what to look for when I was in school, I think it would have helped so many undiagnosed students like myself. I have this type of conversation in a more subtle way with co-workers now that I'm a substitute and work with special needs students, many of whom are autistic.

You just have to know autistic people, you have to be trained to understand what their brain is like. When I was young the symptoms I had were primarily internal within my thought process. I didn't know they were symptoms, and other people certainly didn't know—it was just my normal. Even outward symptoms, like textile sensitivities, where certain fabrics just didn't feel right, were passed off as nothing notable because some materials are just itchy. Textile sensitivity alone wouldn't be a cause for concern, but that in addition to a cluster of other symptoms like how I really disliked loud noises, and my inability to grasp how to put myself in someone else's shoes, drew a broader picture. All of these symptoms that you can now find information on through a few fairly dependable online resources, were symptoms that I didn't know were abnormal to begin with.

Again, if educators had been trained to look for that, they would have noticed when I was very young that something was different. It's not like I was shy about it and wanted to keep all these things to myself. I had no shame about it because I didn't feel I needed to have shame. As far as I knew, everyone else very much disliked loud noises, was task-oriented, and at the age of five was frustrated when someone else did not achieve a desired objective. So those little things like hyper-fixation are like little Easter eggs, little bread crumbs for knowing that you are autistic, but even now a lot of educators, from what I can tell, don't seem to know to look for it.

I work in an inclusive school which means they are obligated and designed to actively incorporate Special Needs students in General Education classrooms, but the teachers are not necessarily required to have extensive special education training. They could be a fully credentialed teacher, teaching a class with five special needs students, one with Down syndrome, three with autism, and one with Oppositional Defiance, but have very little training, if any on how to deal with that.

I've seen it so many times as a sub. Some Special Needs students perform well, get a great deal of accolades, and then are immediately handed more responsibility. It sounds good, but the problem is, they don't have the emotional tools to handle more. That is exactly how it was for me when I was in school. For the Special Needs students that don't perform well, and perhaps demonstrate disruptive behavior, they get punished by points being taken away or being labeled as defiant. They too are not really getting their core emotional, cognitive needs met. In my opinion, when you say inclusive in this manner, it's only on paper, not in practice, because the educators have not been trained to understand what makes the Special Needs students tick. Instead, they are putting Band-Aids over the symptoms.

I'm not trying to criticize the educational system per se, as whatever weakness is there speaks for itself, still, I do believe there is a great deal of room for improvement in this particular area.

Do you think your generation is more plugged in to Special Needs?

My generation is the first generation that really seems to be notably more engaged with this issue. Not all of my generation has kids yet, but the people have heard of autism and seen it represented more, which is a lot more than I had in my childhood. Since they've seen it represented, they are aware of it, aware of the challenges, and aware that it's something they may want to look out for. Not that it's some harmful virus but that it's a condition of living that can be more challenging. Seeing the representation on TikTok, movies, and television, and even medical journals with more nuanced analyses, makes a difference in keeping it in someone's mind, versus how it has been long-neglected in media and research, with some people's main exposure being when they see a kid with some unusual symptoms when they are out and about and they think, *Wow, he's weird,* and then keep going on with their day.

For years, the public wasn't exposed enough to it to think how it might affect someone's life, or wonder if it would affect them. Being a younger parent in this modern time, I think it's much more clearly pragmatic to acknowledge that autism and Special Needs are a possibility. I have talked to some of my close friends that are my age about it, and even though none of us have kids, we are all naturally aware of it because we've grown up around it. We've seen more autistic people and have seen it represented much more, so now it naturally occurs to us to be aware of how we might seek help for a loved one in need. Even though it's possible that plenty of people my age might do a poor job of it because they may not know what to do, at least more people are aware of autism's prevalence and know to do something.

You went away to college only a year or so after finding out you were autistic. What was that like for you?

It was good to learn to be away for the sake of individuality. I think I needed to develop that, especially at that time in my late teens. It was just something I needed to grasp, otherwise it would have been too easy to cling on to whatever I thought my parents wanted me to be, as codependency was natural for me and finding myself was frightening. Going away to college was helpful, but also frustrating in part because of autism and in part just because of people. I didn't love having five roommates because I didn't have space to feel comfortable with myself. My roommate would sleep almost naked and had a scent of old food. As an autistic person you're sensitive to all these different senses, so you don't feel very comfortable when you are consistently with a space, scent, and texture you don't like.

I never felt relaxed or comfortable there. Not that I was particularly stressed out, I just felt out of my element, which of course is rather typical for an autistic person. I didn't know my roommate well, so it's not like we were best friends making a life together or anything like that. I didn't have a car, so everything I did was on campus, and there wasn't a ton to do. That was especially hard as someone who is task-oriented and needed something to do. I had envisioned college to be where I could go out and do something without a specific idea of what those things would be. It was frustrating at times because on weekends, I would go to the gym on campus, come back to my room, listen to a podcast, and just kinda wait for the day to pass by. I imagine that would have been a challenge for any college-age student, but I think being autistic amplified it because there was no *routine* to be built.

Besides not having much to do, I didn't know many people in my classes. For one, I was shy and scarcely talked to people or found them interesting, to be honest. Ironically, when I finally started to socialize, Covid hit, so I never really got to experience "College Life" to fruition.

Since I didn't have a real friend group, and I didn't have the resources in mind to develop one, I would spend long hours browsing online. I went from working long hours at the school newspaper, to doing not much of anything other than making sure my schoolwork was correct, which ended up leading to a lot of frustration as I learned that there were some classes I had taken that were unnecessary. I went over this with my guidance counselors so many times and had specifically asked about taking only the courses I needed, only to find out I had been given incorrect information. It was a lot for me. I felt like I short-circuited. I was only focused on getting the right classes to get my degree and hopefully enjoying myself mildly to moderately, if at all possible.

At first, I had a therapist with whom I spoke on the phone, which was helpful for the initial transition. When you are autistic, you often need extra help reorienting your focus, effort, and your comfort when there is any type of transition or switching from task to task. College was filled with so much transition, it was over-stimulating as I would go from working at the school newspaper to prepping a paper for a class. I also needed significant time to come down from my social brain, which was preoccupied thinking about people's feelings, trying to anticipate the interactions I might have, and instinctively going over what I just said to someone in my head. I would naturally replay it in my mind, how every conversation went and how I could do it differently next time, essentially going through drafts of the interactions.

As I tried to slow down and shift from task to task, I would feel so exhausted from analyzing all the interactions I had. Having a counselor in the beginning really helped take a weight off my shoulders, but I'm also glad that at a certain point I was able to take time away from counseling in order to practice self-soothing.

Seven months into your college experience, Covid hit, and you had to come back home and finish your schooling online. How did that situation affect your sense of self?

Honestly, my sense of self at that point wasn't about me. I was hiding from myself, I was all about trying to get school work done. It was a task I had to complete. I was glad to be home with my parents, but I really wanted to make sure I finished every class so I could finally be done with it all. I was just beginning classes geared toward my interest in TV writing as things went remote. What would have normally come with more individualized passion for me, now came with a sense of uncertainty and obligation. With the shutdown, I couldn't go out and about to diversify my life experiences anyway, so I became consumed with my writing projects.

Fortunately my sense of self wasn't completely on autopilot, it was actually starting to peek through just a bit. I began noticing that I was starting to develop my own personal feelings about my writing. Little by little, I became more proactive in connecting with my online professors and asking for help. I could see traces of individuality shining through but through the task-oriented framework of wanting to get things done. While I was consumed with completing my degree, I was also starting to feel my feelings stronger and clearer than ever before.

If you wrote out a timeline of key points from age eighteen to twenty-three, what would that look like?

At age eighteen, I started therapy and found it very interesting to acknowledge there were issues—low self esteem being a big one—and the most notable event being getting diagnosed as autistic.

At age nineteen, I had my first severe bout with OCD. I didn't know what it was initially, but I could see how serious it was, so I started searching for understanding. I felt extremely relieved when I was officially diagnosed with OCD because it suddenly made a lot of sense. It decreased in intensity for a while, which was helpful because it was just the biggest torture I had ever experienced and had been unable at that point to explain it to anyone.

At age twenty, it was a time of refocusing primarily on my school work, discovering more about myself a little at a time and slowly connecting with others.

At age twenty-one, I began a more substantive OCD work and discovered my bend toward codependency and sought to understand how to navigate through that. It was at this time that I had my first girlfriend. It was an intense seven-month relationship, but it felt notably longer and not because it was a great time. I associate that part of my life with a lot of growth personally because I discovered so much codependency in that relationship. I learned a lot about myself by learning what didn't work with me, and that relationship was quite clearly one of those things that didn't work. Discovering more about codependency and OCD through my lens of autism was huge for my personal development.

Age twenty-two was about grieving. Grief has been described by some as *love that outlives a relationship*. I found grief for the way I treated myself when I was younger and held such low self esteem. I also grieved greatly over my ex-girlfriend who broke up with me in December of 2021. The break-up happened a few days before Christmas. We were on the phone in the morning, and she told me she loved me and wanted to marry me, a sentiment I strongly shared, all the way until she quite abruptly ended the relationship later that day.

One thing I have learned about myself as an autistic person is that it is very difficult for me to let go of commitments I've made. I couldn't comprehend not marrying her once we had already shared that agreement. So a good portion of being twenty-two was me trying to process *how* someone could do that while also learning to accept it.

I started working as a substitute in special education, which helped me feel productive. Even though the work itself was frustrating, I had a tangible understanding of my impact, an embrace of my competence, and an acceptance of the times. When all was said and done, twenty-two was largely about grieving the lies of low self esteem I believed in my youth while learning to embrace adulthood.

Now at twenty-three, I simply and comfortably feel like I have arrived at twenty-three. That is the only reasonable expectation I think I can have. For so long I felt like I had to be at a certain level of maturity, but as I began to discover my life through the lens of autism and self esteem, and navigate through OCD and codependency, I learned the importance of not holding myself to unreasonable standards.

So here I am. I've arrived at twenty-three; I am where I am, and that's cool by me.

As you began to understand your own diagnosis, was it easy or hard to get others closest to you on board in understanding?

I think I tried more when I was younger to get people to

understand, but as I get older, the less I expect them too. I don't mean that in a cynical way, it's just that as I started to grow into understanding myself, the less I held that obligation to others. People around me don't have to understand autism in order to respect my boundaries that are specific to me being autistic. It's the same way that if you don't understand all of Islam, but have a friend who stops answering your texts to pray five times a day, you might glean that prayer time is a special boundary they need as a Muslim. You may be unfamiliar with other rules of Islam, but nevertheless, you give them their space, you understand that boundary, and you respect them.

Similarly, there's not really much accommodation that should happen with OCD, because that's one of the unhealthy things people with OCD rely on. If we are afraid of something we will try and use people as a buffer. For example, if you are afraid of going around a child because you obsessively fear you will hit them, you may ask a friend to go in front of you. That type of accommodation only enables the fear further. It's more of an autistic thing to try and get others to *understand*. With OCD it just might be explaining to someone how you are trying to work through a fear, i.e., *I want to face my fear, can you let me do this?* That's really an easy way to help other people understand where you are, without going in depth about lizard-brain stuff.

I hold myself to a standard of allowing myself to feel secure in my behaviors. As long as other people are considerate, respectful, and demonstrate moral behaviors, then I personally want to prioritize feeling secure in those around me versus having to overly explain myself or apologize for being autistic. That is very often the context in which people explain their autism, as if there is a deficiency and they just want to make sure others understand why they are so lackluster. But for me it's really a matter of now knowing I feel appropriate to my environment, I can ask for something if I need it, and if someone has a problem with how I ask for it, they can approach me, and we can resolve it together. Now having that basic fundamental skill, if someone thinks I am coming across sharp or blunt, which is often associated with high-functioning autism, and they tell me, then it is something we can definitely resolve. In that context I may offer an apology and let them know I'm autistic and didn't realize I was coming across that way. On the other hand, if they don't tell me, I can't hold myself to the standard of reading their mind.

Did you hear the phrase, "But you don't seem autistic" a lot?

Oh yeah. From what I can tell, when people hear autism, they seem to envision Down syndrome, even though it's an entirely different thing altogether. I think the notion of having physical traits of autism or *sounding* autistic is what some people tend to think of as someone who speaks slowly or with a strange cadence, but it is not necessarily true. It's been easier for me over time to not try and convince people I'm autistic, as if there is a need to justify or validate my own existence. It's really not their job to understand me or my job to convince them. Sometimes random people have come out and *told* me, "Well, you are low on the spectrum." They assert it as fact. I don't take offense to it much anymore. Someone may choose to understand what being autistic is, if they want, but if someone says, *Oh you're not "really" autistic*, it just shows me that they're not that inclined to learn, and I'm not trying to force someone to learn when they don't want to, because that would be frustrate me for no good reason.

You work with special needs kids, many who are diagnosed as autistic, do you find yourself identifying with them?

I very much identify with a lot of the things the autistic students experience even though I didn't share their specific symptoms when I was younger. The fundamental mechanisms are very similar. Their feeling exceptionally agitated when they're overstimulated is so relatable. There have been times I've heard sounds that I just hate, and it makes me want to punch someone in the face. Not because I'm mad at them, but because it's an extreme sensitivity, and it bothers me so much that my thoughts in those moments are along the lines of, *Get out of my face.* You just need that space.

It could be the most benign sound, but if it doesn't feel right to the kids I work with they will freak out, and I so understand. I just happened to have more impulse control fortunately to not freak out as a child, but I felt the strong frustration and the urge to just break something like they do. It lets out a lot of adrenaline, which can help you feel in control.

It still pops up randomly for me, and I'll be surprised by it. It could be the smallest sound, but it immediately agitates me.

Fortunately, I now have a wonderful girlfriend who is really understanding. If she happens to make a sound or a noise even jokingly that I find I'm extremely sensitive to, I just let her know that I'm struggling, and she has really surprised me with how understanding she is.

Gaining a sense of self can be challenging for anyone, but as you observe the special needs students you work with would you say it's a bit harder when you are on the spectrum?

I think it is a bit harder for them to gain a sense of self, because people around them are often trying to manage their symptoms by containing them, instead of facilitating their well-being by helping them understand themselves and express themselves in healthier ways.

For example, aides and teachers may give an autistic student a treat to stop a tantrum or pacify them in general because they don't want them to bother the class, whereas facilitating their well-being might mean bringing them to a room where they can calm down for fifteen minutes and then walking them back to class and letting them try for five seconds to just sit down before bringing them back out of the room then trying that again and again throughout the day.

It varies a lot, but Special Ed kids often require certain accommodations; they fundamentally *need* it in order to operate at the level teachers expect other students to.

When you were in school you were not perceived as a special needs student but rather as a gifted student recommended for a number of high performing programs. Now, in retrospect, what do you think you needed at that time?

I think I personally would have been better suited for a G.E. class with drop in assistance. I didn't need the constant prompting to do work or to go from transition to transition because I knew how to follow along, but it would have been beneficial in my view if I had not only understood that I was on the spectrum, but if I had a counselor or aide drop in regularly to see how I was doing and invite me to express my needs in the classroom.

At one of the schools where I was a sub, I worked with some middle of the road special needs students who just needed a bit of help with their emotional and verbal skills. We would use a token board as an easy way to invite these students to express their feelings and to encourage them to advocate for themselves. A tool like a token board when you are autistic can help a lot because you are able to build a positive association with things you don't understand or dislike instead of responding with sheer negative impulse. If there had been this type of tool for me when I was young, I know I would have benefited greatly.

Writing has been a way of expression and a good outlet for you since you were little. Now in hindsight, do you think writing helped you even more being that you were autistic and didn't know?

For sure. When I was younger, I found writing validating and comforting. I would often write about things that irritated me, small frustrations, things I was inflexible about. It was something that I think if I had done more of and had the infrastructure around me in the educational setting, a counselor or teacher would have been able to quickly notice my emotional process. I think they might have noticed that I hyper-fixated on certain interests across all of my writings, or that I had an inability to understand other people's motivations or feelings—again, all little bread crumbs for autism.

I think it was helpful to express it, for at least setting a small one-word blueprint of what expression meant to me. Having that record of writing reminds me that I can share thoughts and feelings in this format now.

In terms of now, I write about characters having things I can relate to like OCD and autism. I recently wrote a feature length film about a homicide journalist with OCD. One of the difficulties I found in writing the script was trying to explain OCD. At first I was looking for a way to explain it without banging people over the head with it, but I realized people kind of have to be banged over the head with it a bit to help them understand such a foreign idea. It's not like people are trying to be ignorant, they just don't know. Having this little niche of things is nice for me.

I don't usually enjoy making the standard cop dramas, because I know where they are going, and I don't have an attachment to any of the characters. But if I can create something kind of tonally niche against a backdrop of what broader audiences enjoy, it makes me feel less isolated from people who connect to things that I don't. Some of the things I'm more confident to write about now are OCD and autism. Another script that I still have to finish has an autistic character in Western Expansion. Even though people have been autistic for generations, they just really haven't been included in history for consideration, so it's nice to make a narrative where I can see myself.

As an autistic person with OCD, over-thinking and over-calculating has been an issue for you in the past. How do you manage that now that you understand more about yourself?

There is this theory known as *Occam's Razor Theory*, which originated with philosophers years ago and has since become a common cog in problem solving. It asserts, "The simplest solution is most often the correct one." For me, in trying to manage my very particular brain, I *try* to go for the simplest solution so I don't get overwhelmed. Now I tend to reserve calculating in a positive way for the sake of achieving a specific goal and prospering professionally. It's easier for me now as I recognize my own competence, and therefore don't really feel as much of a need to calculate in order to appeal to people like I used to.

I know doing well at work and earning money is very important to you as well as to most people, but would you say earning money is a hyper-fixation for you?

It's definitely an area that's important to me and it's something I could curb, but it's difficult when I know it's also pragmatically important for living life. It is probably something I think about more than my peers. I was out with my friends the other day. We went to Applebee's and I was hesitant to pay for an eight-dollar drink, even though I have over ten thousand dollars in my account. We split the tab but my friend initially put it on her card. However, she checked her bank account first to make sure she had enough money to cover the bill. I could never think of doing that. I would never *want* to be in a position where I had to check to make sure I had enough for at least a meal. I have constant awareness, a vigilance to grow financially. I wouldn't say it's a hyper-fixation, but there is definitely added pressure because of my tendency to ruminate more.

You chose to address both OCD and codependency head on, which was harder and was it worth it?

The fact that I'm better off as a person means I can objectively say, yes, all the hard work has been worth it. I feel healthier and self-sufficient knowing I can accomplish whatever I set my mind to. I'm more confident now that I can meet my own basic needs, or as Nathaniel Branden says in his book *The Six Pillars of Self Esteem*, I can see my own self-efficacy.

Just noting that you have the capability, physically and mentally, to take care of your own basic needs is often lost on people with low self esteem, which is a common comorbidity for an autistic people. Finally getting to a place of understanding that you really can take care of yourself, earn a living, and be a productive person in society despite immense doubt, is absolutely amazing.

In terms of which was harder, I couldn't tell you. I would have to say pick your poison. OCD is like an acute pain where you have just been punched in the face, and codependency is more like a slow choke—both comparable and seemingly unbearable pains.

The greatest thing in coming through at least the starting point of codependency and OCD treatment was realizing, *Oh, I actually have a say in this.* I liken it to video games, where there are characters you can't play or change known as non-playable characters or NPCs. Understanding myself as a person on the spectrum and learning to manage OCD and codependency helped me know that I'm not an NPC, or a nonfactor in my own life. I actually lead it. So yes, I would say it's worth it; not that it's been easy because nothing so worthwhile is easy, but it is definitely worth it.

Goals seem to be a key topic for you. Why is that?

I find setting and meeting goals very fulfilling. For some people it's social relationships, meeting new people, going on vacations. But for me, I personally like achieving things. I imagine this interest of achieving whatever goal I choose is influenced by autism, but there are also a lot of goal-oriented people out there that are not autistic at all—it's just what they like. One thing I have learned is that the way I go about achieving a goal can definitely lead to hyper-fixation, but the goal itself, I like. It helps me feel structured and enthused.

One of my goals at the moment is to bulk up a bit. Thankfully, it's not because I dislike how I look or that I think I'm unappealing, as I thought for years. It's just something I get to enjoy doing for me.

On a deeper level, another goal is to continue learning to accept—accept what I'm thinking, what I'm feeling, and accepting uncertainty, which is a huge thing for OCD. It's just a matter of knowing that I'm right here, I'm good, and submitting to reality will bring me more peace in the long run.

Since you have reached a point of not needing to explain yourself as being on the spectrum to anyone, what would you say is the main point for doing this book?

This book is an opportunity for people to learn a bit about what it is like being on the autism spectrum, at least for me, and the value of hindsight where that is concerned. People *choosing* to read this book sets a more open-minded tone than me trying to force unsolicited information on them. But also, a big part of this book is about me having the courage within myself to openly share my own complicated feelings and hopefully encourage others to do the same.

As a young man in his early twenties, Isaiah is still discovering his overall sense of self, but in the last five years since learning he was on the spectrum and all that it entails, he has grown by leaps and bounds and has developed such a solid sense of who he is, which I can't say he would have done quite the same way if he hadn't gone through some of his experiences.

I'm not sure how other parents would feel if they were told their child was on the spectrum at eighteen. I would imagine some might feel angry, maybe relieved, or confused as to why they didn't know earlier. We certainly had a range of our own emotions and thoughts about it all, but I can honestly say now that all those feelings are valid. As parents, we want to be in the know at all times when it comes to our kids, and we want the best for them. But when it comes to something like this, whether you find out earlier or later, I think the most important thing is to process the information the best you know how and move forward with an accepting mind and a willing heart. That's the best thing any parent can do when it comes to their kids, spectrum or not.

Isaiah would have most definitely benefited by knowing he was autistic when he was younger, which would perhaps have led to the extra support that he needed—but he didn't have such a diagnosis. One thing he did have was a God-given gift for writing. I recall when he was in first grade, there was a little girl who was not being very nice to him. I'm not sure if she actually had a crush on him or not, but she was a li'l stinker towards him, or better said, a big stinker. Isaiah never told me of the issue or expressed his feelings and frustrations about it. Knowing what I know now about autism, I realize he was unable to verbally express those kinds of things, but he was able to write a fiction story, and that's how I learned there was a problem with a little girl in his class. So while God saw fit, for His reasonings, to wait on revealing Isaiah's diagnosis, He also saw fit to provide Isaiah the gift of writing to allow a decent measure of expression.

What I have learned most over the last five years is that people, including myself at one point, really have a limited understanding about the autism spectrum, OCD, and a slew of other mental health disorders. While there may be some similarities in each disorder, as you can see from Isaiah's story, everyone experiences it a little bit differently.

Isaiah was an adult when he received his diagnosis, and he didn't have a lot of resources to pull from, but thankfully, he opted to do the adult thing and address his diagnosis in ways that would best help him understand his own self in order to help him grow. Obviously as his mom, if I could have taken some of the struggle away from him, I would have; but I couldn't. Whether as an autistic person, or simply my son, there have just been some things that he had to walk through by himself because trying to do it for him would have only enabled him. So while mama is always nearby, he is navigating his life on the spectrum and in general, one step at a time and doing a fine job of it.

"But now, O Lord, you are our Father; we are the clay, and you are our potter; we are all the work of your hand."
—Isaiah 64:8

PART IV

Retrospect

Mom:

Isaiah and I just had an enlightening conversation that really sums up the reason for this book.

When all the questions had been asked and answers given, I asked Isaiah to write the Introduction and Final Thoughts for Part IV being that it was filled with his question for me.

For the introduction, I asked Isaiah to write about his thoughts on doing this book with me and why he chose the questions he chose for me. And for his final thoughts, I asked him to write how he felt about having the question and answer time with me, elaborating even more as to why he chose the questions he chose, and finally, adding how doing this book together and sharing openly feels for him.

Isaiah took his time to thoughtfully write out both sections that I requested and then emailed it to me last night so that I could include what he wrote in the final manuscript.

Now I am fully aware that our styles of writing vary greatly. I tend to think he writes like a grown up with big words, many of which I literally have to look up the definition for; where I myself tend to be more of a *See Spot Run* kind of writer. Regardless of our different styles, I assumed that because this book is a joint effort, our different styles would mesh together for the sake of *Autism in Hindsight*. I assumed that Isaiah would send me what he had written and that I would be able to copy and paste it right into the manuscript with ease.

However, that wasn't exactly the case. When I read through what Isaiah wrote, it surprisingly stopped me in my tracks. To be honest, I wasn't sure I understood all of what he was saying, and I didn't know how to respond or what I was feeling about it all.

I have made every effort to allow Isaiah to speak freely (when we were recording) without taking his answers personally or taking them to heart in such a way that it might become a hindrance. But with his written words for the final section and the kind of questions he asked me, I found myself questioning if I am truly understanding my son and where he is in his life's journey. I was also momentarily consumed with how I could blend his writing a bit to flow best with the book. Should I cut it? Rewrite it? While contemplating those things, my own mama insecurities popped up as I read his words. Maybe to an outsider, there was nothing that would seem to be a reason for insecurity, but for me, the mom who raised three kids alongside my husband, there was a bit of a trigger.

Fortunately, I have had enough experience with Isaiah to know that I could sit down and ask him for clarity, and he would give it.

As we talked through his Intro and Final Thoughts along with the questions he had asked me, Isaiah explained to me yet again, that "Autism is a disorder where you chronically seek order, that's the irony of the whole thing."

He has explained this in different ways many times over the last few years since being diagnosed, but because my thought process is so different and because I viewed him differently for so long, I've needed a lot of reminders along the way.

When it came to the questions he asked, it helped him in finding his own order and understanding as a person, let alone as an autistic person because he was learning about my background in certain areas.

When it came to writing the Intro and Final Thoughts the way he did, Isaiah explained that he was free writing the very things that allowed him to connect dots from being an undiagnosed autistic child to becoming a diagnosed autistic young man. In free writing he admits he wasn't focused on the book, *Autism in Hindsight,* he was simply focused on expressing what he felt in the moment as an autistic person, and what he felt was clarity. He reiterated the need to understand the behind the scenes information to us as his parents, to our family, in order to better process his world.

Then with a grin he added:

"Ironically, what this book is about and what happened with this conversation is that, I'm autistic. I perceive things differently and so when you read my writing, that was me perceiving things differently and you perceiving things differently than me, which is fine, we just needed to understand—which is what the whole book is about."

In the midst of us both laughing at the irony, he added, *"This could very well be the last scene of the book."*

With that said, with the exception of a line or two, I opted for leaving Isaiah's writing as is and allowing readers to draw their own conclusion, or better yet, choose to understand why this just might be a perfect example for this book.

ISAIAH:

"You're in danger," I heard, in the form of a hot flow of blood swishing in my chest. Call it temporary palpitations or a mild case of the heebie-jeebies, but fear was instinctive. Both on an innate biological level and through a learned pathology of fretful anticipation, my response to even the most minute of unknowns can be hyper-vigilance.

All my mother had said was, "Hey, so…" as her eyes trailed off and she chewed her lip in contemplation. My brain scarcely *hears* silence. More often, it hears what it believes will come next. An innocent, "Hey, so…" was filtered through my perception as "Hey, so we're kicking you out the house because you forgot to do something we asked you to do the other day, you scraped my car, and you got three girls pregnant." While I hadn't done any of those things, my (well-intending) brain was making up things to worry about because it was looking for an excuse to keep me safe and preempt any possible threat. That's great…when there's an actual threat. It's less conducive to a productive conversation when the threat is hypothetical, yet treated as real, and the whole time, my mother was only working to verbalize some form of, "Hey, so… I have this idea for this book. Would you be alright if I interviewed you for it?"

Some at even a stereotypical level are likely familiar with pattern recognition as a hallmark of autism. For some autistic individuals, it may be the pursuit of assigning numerical values to each step of the Hero's Journey in one's favorite Young Adult novel. For others, it's memorizing sports statistics, obscure religious lore, trading card games; what have you. The common thread of these hyper-fixations is the individual's ability to self-regulate by engaging in these interests. Their happy place might not only be a place, but a set of facts, ideas, and symbols.

Who cares? Well, autistic people. Why? I dunno. I don't

share most of those interests. I only mention it because one of the most notable hyper-fixations I've noticed in myself has been social behavior. Meticulous calculations to calibrate my voice, my attire, my posture, and my word-choice were made in a scrounging attempt to feel appropriate to my surroundings. At a young age, it simply felt like a natural, unspoken necessity to me. Even into my early twenties, I was a child mimicking people who I thought had a superior understanding of life.

Beethoven went deaf after a while. Fun fact. Unless you're Beethoven. He suffered a fundamental disconnect from the service he was providing to audiences. But he still made music. A rough feeling from the vibrations of the music he composed, paired with a recollection of how notes would theoretically sound together, were all that bolstered him while he wrote what would become his more famous pieces. Somewhat comparably, I could relate to the idea of wanting to achieve something great while feeling that an innate divide kept me from fully connecting to others. The main difference being, however, that while Beethoven spent his efforts to thrive in making history-defining music. I exerted far less self-assured efforts just trying to justify my own existence.

Struggling to understand which traits of mine were just "autistic things" and which weren't, I started seeing my parents through a different lens. It wasn't quite geared toward blaming them for the way I was or the choices I'd made, but more of a sobering study to see how far the apple had fallen from the tree. If my family tree comprised a TV show, I felt like I started watching during season five and could benefit from a "Previously On" segment. I already knew who was in the good books and the bad, whose parents had cheated on whom, and why so-and-so was mad about something from 1996. I just didn't know the emotional toll many things took on my mom. So I looked for the most pertinent personal questions I could find. *NY Times' 36 Questions to Fall in Love* had a few to offer. I reworded some and came up with a few of my own, and felt that the small handful of questions that came of it would ultimately draw an intimate portrait of not only the woman who raised me, but more notably, the young girl she sought to heal.

"Sometimes the things we can't change end up changing us"

–Unknown

Talking with Mom

What do you notice about yourself in hindsight?

I've noticed many things about myself in hindsight, but I would have to say one of the major things I have noticed about myself is how codependency has been a struggle for almost all of my entire life.

Just like when you told me that codependency felt normal to you and that you didn't know it was an unhealthy thing until you did, that's exactly how I felt as well. And I only learned about it when you were barely a teenager, so not that long ago. I had no idea what codependency was prior to that and how my own upbringing developed that side of me. Being codependent was such a significant part of my life, and I thought it was completely normal until I learned otherwise.

Initially when I first started hearing about this term, "codependent," I wanted to point fingers at other people, but as I continued to learn, especially when reading the same book you eventually read, *Codependent No More* by Melody Beattie, I began to understand that I needed to address some issues within myself. It's still a journey I work through. I would have to say it is probably the biggest thing that has impacted who I am as a person and how I operate in both good and bad ways.

What I have learned about myself in this area is that there is always this thin line I can easily cross over. One side of the line is being genuinely concerned about the well being of those closest to me, wanting to support them however I can which really is a good quality. However, the other side of the line is me taking on responsibilities that are not mine to take on at all. It's trying to overly help and overly fix things to a fault, things that were never meant for me to take on, things that only end up enabling others if I'm not careful. That has been the challenge.

In hindsight, I look back and think, *Wow if I had always known about the unhealthy nature of codependency, that really would have impacted how I was in key relationships like with my children, my spouse, my mom and so on.* If I had actually understood that whole concept about codependency then, and how to navigate through it, accepting my own responsibilities and allowing others to do the same, I would have been a completely different person. Not necessarily better or worse, but definitely different. Though I learned about all this later in life, I'm still very glad because I'm growing into a different person now. Navigating that fine line will probably be a lifelong journey for me, but I'm okay with that. To be honest, I feel proud of myself whenever I recognize that I'm responding to a circumstance or situation in a much healthier, non-codependent way.

If you could go back in time, what would you change about how you were raised?

That's a great question. If I could go back and change something, having the insight that I have now, I would definitely have to say that it would be the codependent issues that I picked up from my parents' relationship. Not to knock my parents in anyway because I love them greatly and believe with all my heart that they did the very best they knew how as parents, but if I could have somehow understood when I was little, which is so difficult to do as a child, that I am not responsible for their decisions, that would have been incredible. If I had understood that I was not responsible for their deceptions, for their divorce, for my mom's heartache after the divorce and poor choices made based on insecurity. If I had somehow known how to let my parents carry their own baggage and not have felt the need to carry it for them, that would have been a complete game-changer for me.

I think I knew deep down on some level that I wasn't really responsible for their choices, but in practice I could just name countless of times, basically all of my life that my inner struggles, the inner turmoil I had was because I was feeling responsible for somebody else's feelings and not having a clue about my own.

Coming into that understanding as an adult, although definitely better late than never, is still a challenge, but I'm getting there. Sometimes my thoughts are like, *Man oh man, that would have helped so much to have this understanding then.* Most of the struggles in this area stemmed from the relationship with my mom, but certainly it wasn't like she was trying to put that codependent thing on me. It was her own insecurities, her own life, her own way, and then not knowing herself as well as she may have thought she did. I was raised feeling one hundred percent responsible for her feelings whether she realized it or not.

Like I said, there is this fine line. Sometimes I look at it and realize God made me the kind of person to actually care about other people deeply, to be really tuned into people, but now I understand the difference between how God made me caring versus my bent toward codependency.

Now I can tell when I'm being mindful of God's nudge to help someone versus me just taking up responsibility for somebody and trying to help or fix in a way that I was never meant to do. I definitely haven't mastered the whole thing, and it sure does stink when all of a sudden I realize I'm operating in that codependent way again, but those are few and far between now as I most definitely can see so much more clearly.

In one sentence, how would you describe from your point of view, codependency?

From my point of view, codependency is feeling one hundred percent responsible for someone else's happiness and well-being and just their overall feelings. It really is like you mentioned that feeling of, *I'm not okay if you're not okay.*

For me, when someone close to me needs my help and I'm able to help them then everything feels good and balanced, but if they're struggling, especially with their emotions, it's extremely hard for me to just be okay. I'll have an edgy, uncomfortable, anxious feeling in my gut until I know things have shifted to what's normal for me. That might sound as if I'm being intuitive, and sometimes it is. But if I'm not careful, that thin line gets crossed over and quickly turns unhealthy for me.

I find that the people I can get most codependent with are the ones who seek me out for attention and really pursue my help, which again isn't necessarily bad in itself, but when I don't pay attention, I can easily find myself on the wrong side of that thin line. Before you know it, I'm the fixer, the mediator, the problem-solver and more to a situation that really doesn't involve me, or at least doesn't need to. It's a crazy cycle. One I'm very glad to be growing through.

You've talked about how you were raised and how you raised me, which both seemed to bookend this period that you've described as oblivion. You were just living life, trying to deal with stuff, but slowly came to this realization of why you felt the way you did and operated the way you did. With that said, how does your realizing things for yourself tie together in raising me?

By the time you came along, I had already had a lot of crazy life experiences. A truly significant turning point for me, however, was when I came to a place of discovering God in a personal way, becoming a Christian and actually applying God's Word to my life. Discovering that God wasn't just *the man upstairs* as I had often heard Him referred to as, but instead God was real and was with me, and honestly changed me from the inside out. It was at that point that I understood there was a whole other life for me as a person in Christ. Of course all of that did not make my codependent nature go away, but it sure connected a lot of dots for me with life, my overall identity, and who I was just as a person in general.

Naturally, everybody goes through that point of where they initially identify with the family that raises them, but then you grow up a bit and actually develop your own identity. I found my identity in Jesus. As I started learning about His unconditional love and how He actually has a specific plan for everyone's life, and how He understands literally everything about us because He created us, my life started changing. That change didn't start happening until I was almost thirty.

Then you came along about five years later. By that time, so much of my identity was in my growing relationship with Jesus and what the Bible actually said about me. For example, I grew up feeling insecure, but the Bible taught me that I am secure in Christ. Learning those things and understanding how the way I viewed myself really didn't have to be set in stone based on all the circumstances of my life but in what God's word says about me and about all of us really.

I had been processing those things for a while, and it's not that I felt like I had arrived, but I felt like I had a solid understanding of who I was in God, and I felt I was so much better for it.

Then you came along. As you are very familiar with the story, God put you on my heart and spoke to my spirit, not in an audible voice but in a knowing, letting me know that I was to pray for you, my unborn son, which I did for five years before you showed up on the scene. For me it felt like you were there long before you were born, and by then I felt like I was a solid person of faith, believing in God's hand in my life every day and all that good faith-filled stuff. I thought once you were born, I would raise you in faith and assumed it would be non-complicated.

But I eventually realized I still had a lot of unhealthy residue in me. Yes, I was a believer, and God was working in me and through me one day at a time, but there was still a lot of emotional, PTSD-ish kinda stuff to work through.

Like I've said, I was already on that journey of self discovery, but it was a long time for those journeys. I was already thirty-five when you were born, and by the time I read *Codependency No More* and really started to understand my codependent nature, I was in my forties. I was raising you guys in faith, yes, while still getting little bits and pieces of understanding of my own way of doing things.

Honestly, one of the reasons why I was even interested in putting this book together and thought it was such a neat idea to write a bit about this journey of yours was because I know how as a young person it wasn't an easy ride for you. You ended up addressing things for yourself at a young age that I didn't even know to address within myself until I was twice your age.

You were only twenty-two when you did the NOCD program, and that was the most challenging thing ever. Out of all the stuff you were learning about yourself from being on the autism spectrum and what that looked like, and then recognizing your own struggle with codependency which affected how you operated, to eventually understanding the reality of your OCD, that was the scariest thing for you.

For me as your mom to see you get to a point where you were so sick of what you didn't even fully understand but willingly sought out help for was incredible. It was difficult to watch you sit with your clearly uncomfortable feelings in order to process your healing. Watching you go through that seemed a lot scarier than my codependent issues. Not that I'm negating my own experiences, but I saw you, and I thought, *Wow, here you are confronting these things out of your need for a healthy survival at a young age and I'm more than twice your age and still learning.* I know you are still learning too, but it encouraged me to see that you kind of knew what to do, or should I say, you willingly learned what to do, which oftentimes was simply being okay with being uncomfortable.

For me to learn that sometimes I have to sit with being

uncomfortable in not operating from a codependent way and trying to fix something, not taking on responsibility for those closest to me—it's been hard. It's much better now, but it has still been hard.

I remember when I was first learning about all this codependent stuff. I had many fears over the fact that I could not control my teenage daughter's choices. I was so worried about where her decisions might lead her, and I just wanted to fix it. I called my best friend in a panic as usual and said, *What if my daughter makes bad choices and dies somewhere out there?* My wise friend briefly paused and then gave this gentle response, *Yes, what if she does?*

I felt so angry when she said that. I thought, *Wait, this is not what my best friend is supposed to say to me. She should tell me not to worry, she should tell me how to save my daughter from her teenage self and she should most definitely fix my feelings.* But she did none of that. Instead, my dearest friend let me sit in the reality of my worst fear for just a bit while she quietly stayed on the other end of the line.

That was one of the first times that I really sat with my feelings, and although I was scared, in truth it helped me. It was at that moment where my best friend, who also happened to be a counselor, didn't enable my codependent behavior.

In that moment, I recognized just how much my codependent nature ruled me. Thankfully because I had a growing faith-filled relationship with God, I began praying about how to break free from codependency and sought my own help and continue to do so. As you have stated, some of your codependent nature was learned from me early on, but fortunately both of us have held ourselves accountable and have grown better for it.

If you could go back and change one thing about how you raised me, what would that be?

Wow! Another great question. My first thought was saying something along the lines of, if I had known myself better then maybe I would have dealt with things a little bit differently, not so much with you, Isaiah, because you were the last child, so I had figured out a thing or two by then. But perhaps with your two older sisters. I was often very reactive in my approach when raising them.

But to be honest, I really was in the process of knowing myself better even when raising them, it just took a while. Since I was already on my journey of self-discovery and healing, I was no longer completely oblivious, but as you well know just because you are on a healing journey doesn't mean you're not gonna have a bad period of time or come unglued a bit before self correcting.

Mostly, I feel that I raised you in a way that I sincerely believed was right. There was always lots of love and my desire was to have closeness, and good communication with all of us as family, but I also realize I'm looking at it from one perspective. I guess the obvious thing I would want to go back and change if I could was knowing that you were autistic early on. None of us knew, but if we had, perhaps we could have helped you communicate and process things in a way that would have benefited you more. At the same time, it's kind of hard to say that, because I've seen you grow into this incredible young man through all of your own experiences, so who's to say how it would have turned out if I had changed things.

As a parent this is how I judge it. I look at all my children, and yes, we had issues just like any other family, but as adults, now that everybody's accountable for themselves, I look at all of you, and I see you all are doing really well. You all care about your own growth mentally, physically, spiritually and continue to strive in those areas, you all make an effort to live genuine and productive lives, and you all really care about other people and desire to make a positive impact.

I see and know the heart of each of you. You're all different, but all of you have a strong foundation, a strong core of belief, and strong, beautiful hearts. I am genuinely proud of how you three have turned out. And while no parent can take all the credit on what kind of adults their kids turn into, I look at you guys and realize that despite the things that were challenging, from codependency tendencies, rebellious spirits, or being on the spectrum without knowing to name a few, as parents we must have done something right, because you all turned out wonderfully.

So with that said, if I could go back and change some things about how I raised you, I might tweak a few things that would make communication smoother, but overall, I wouldn't change too much at all.

What is the biggest thing you don't know but wish you did?

That's kind of a hard question, but I guess it would be to know a little bit of the future in regards to how things all play out.

For example, as we've talked about my codependency nature still rearing up at certain times and me working through it, it would be nice to know how it really all plays out. And maybe know how things play out within our family. I've always had an idea in my head, especially when you guys were little, and things were simple, at least from my point of view. I had such an image in my head of what our family would look like, the dynamics, just the whole thing, you know. We are absolutely a great family and love each other very much, but how I had pictured things when you all were little versus now that everyone is grown is a little different.

I think of the example of how I prayed for you for five years before you were ever born. Knowing all the conversations I had with God and what I felt He was putting on my heart at the time and then to see all these different struggles you've had, I'm like, *Hey God, you didn't tell me that this was going to be a part of it. I wasn't informed.* Of course you have turned out absolutely fine, and I've learned to trust God through it all, but I kind of wished I would have known a few things ahead of time so I could have better helped.

One thing I learned from you when you talked about OCD because the nature of it you said, *This isn't something that completely goes away or you just fix it, but you learn to manage it.* I believe your counselor originally told you that, and it made me think about a lot of things we deal with that don't instantly get fixed. You learn to manage it and grow through it, and over time it becomes much less of an issue. You learn to deal with things productively, in a good way, in a healthy way, and you are able to move forward. I think a lot of life is like that, you know. So in regard to the question you asked, *What is the biggest thing I don't know but wish I did?* It might be nice to know a little bit of the future and how things play out overall, but as long as I know that we all are willing to work through and manage this life God has given us, and trust Him in the process, then I suppose I already know what I need to know.

A "front" isn't necessarily a facade. It's a form of social display, often employed with some degree of emotional distancing. In hindsight, a struggle I faced with my parents was their use of fronts. The "united front," the "disciplined front," the "religious front"—different ways they presented themselves to advocate for different values. It wasn't necessarily bad, but it was invulnerable. Not until some time into my career in education did I begin to recognize something similar in my own experience: I had to find a balance in the amount of vulnerability I was willing to show while assuming an authority role.

For me, it was a difficult balance that I was constantly having to recalibrate through trial and error. With special needs and behavioral needs students, physical safety was an exceptionally common cause for concern. At what I'd like to believe was my most effective state as an educator, I found myself giving each child the benefit of the doubt, but holding steadfast with rules and boundaries when deciding that they are a threat to other students' well-being or unnecessarily disruptive to my job. At my least effective, I worked through fear. I didn't want to be trampled over by twenty-plus ten-year-olds with abusive families and personality disorders. I operated with a motto of "suppress any fires that rise," rather than "engage with troubled students to better understand their behaviors while still expecting quality choices of them."

But I had a privilege that I reveled in everyday—I got to leave. I got to leave the kids I had for that school day, I got to leave the problems of my job at the door, and I got to leave for an environment in which I could comfortably be alone. This space, along with my students not being my flesh and blood, helped immensely in reminding me not to take failures and perceived transgressions personally. It helped me not to have such a "guard up" with each student, so to speak. I'd get close and give them chances and sometimes be disappointed, but never felt foolish for giving them the chance to make a good choice.

Back to the point at hand, I recall talking to my mother, who was musing on the challenges during the teen years when it came to raising my older siblings. In hindsight, I'd say my parents were taking it personally. I mentioned that for much of that decade, my mother and father seemed primarily bitter above all else, especially with household disorder. I was surprised that she didn't contest the label in the slightest. She agreed adamantly. Difficulties from the turbulent teen years with my siblings had left something of a bitter taste in their mouth, even though they deeply loved both my siblings. A common aversion to vulnerability meant that authority picked up the slack in what might have more ideally been a balance. For both of us to hear this from one another was beautifully jarring, especially when so clearly articulated through feelings that were amorphous for so long.

Being told, "We treated you as if you were going to have the same challenges as your siblings, but it turned out you didn't," made all the sense in the world. Their guard was up. They were terrified, but they were trying to love me in as productive a way as possible. But in that moment, there was clearly no "front" to be had in the form of rules or expectations. There wasn't a regimen to which I was being accustomed, but a three-dimensional mutual relationship I was able to discover with my parents through vulnerability and empathy.

As we get closer to the end of this book, I am so very grateful for the challenge and complete joy of discussing autism, OCD, codependency, and the growing pains in between with each other and then sharing it with you, the wonderful reader.

It is hard to communicate at times, for all of us. Often it's not for a lack of desire but because we just don't always understand our own self let alone anyone else, which can make real, honest communication rather difficult.

For my son and I to speak truthfully and respectfully with each other about all that we have learned in hindsight thus far, has been beyond incredible. It's nothing short of God's hand, if you ask me.

If you, dear reader, are a parent and have never considered interviewing your adult child, I would highly recommend it. And if you do, be prepared for a few tears in the midst of many "ah ha" moments.

I would suggest you create a long list of questions, anything you can think of, including those questions you believe you already know the answers to. Then bring your list of questions to your adult child, ask one at a time and then listen, truly listen. You will find that you love much of what you hear and some of what you don't. However, if you create a safe space for your adult child to speak freely and honestly, you will definitely learn so much more about who they are, and they will learn about you, and you both will be immeasurably blessed.

Asking Isaiah the many questions that are shared in this

book as well as many other questions that are not shared here whether it be about the spectrum, anxiety, or life in general has helped me to really understand him in a deeper way—to understand him from his point of view instead of just my own.

My job as Isaiah's mama when he was little was to raise him well and teach him good things. While I was not perfect in any way, I do believe I did my job well. Now that he is an adult, and our roles have changed, we both have learned to communicate with one another on a whole other level. Whether it's about being on the autism spectrum, the intricacies of relationships, goals and dreams, the horrendous fear that unaddressed OCD generates, or life in general, we are teaching each other by growing and learning to be our most honest selves.

Poems, Song, and a Word from Isaiah

TRYING

In loving me, I notice my heart flutters like a broken wing
It aches with every stroke against the wind
Blundering, but prospering nonetheless

–Isaiah Cane

Them

Their words were like poetry. They made no sense.
                                    –Isaiah Cane

Preface

This song I wrote represented a few things to me, but as time has passed, it most notably represents me mourning. More than me lamenting a breakup, I was sobered and at times saddened by the realization that what broke us up was my decision to make healthier choices and her decision to stay the same. I changed the rules. Through a mix of what I'm sure is a thousand quotes in my subconscious, I rendered that grief is love that outlives a relationship. I told my ex this in one of our few interactions post-breakup. It's the only time I can remember her being speechless. While the memory was long tender to the touch, I was still somewhat grateful to have any feeling about it at all. Thus, I wrote—

Good, Grief

Sometimes it feels like post-traumatic Stockholm syndrome. Daily achings for the devil and the sins that got me with him. It's drama, but I'm prompted to err on the side of caution. For too long, my deepest longings were long-forgotten. And you are your father's daughter, so I know you felt no option while trapped within your trauma bond.

No matter how much he gave you then, that now you got, he's always got you hurting over what you're not: Enough for him to love himself. Self-love brought on compunction; an innately destructive function.

For 20-some years this song and dance kept you in a soulless trance. Somehow I met you at this juncture and boils of grief became ready to rupture.

You shared that while you were jiving and grooving one way, you barely evaded an era of "Gloomy Sundays." You swore y'all were moving forward, but maturation isn't linear. That's just another lesson I couldn't force into ya.

And truly, I had no such interest in our early ages. Part of my appeal was how I helped you stay complacent. Unhealthy as we were, I felt no need to send complaints in. This was till the crucial moment I was clutched-chest. Psychosomatic unrest of heat and tingles. Forced to the surface neglected evils.

It began the end of our folie a deux-type love fest. That night, my cross to bear had broke my back. It was a source of pride I needed saving from, in fact. Courage from loving you in some way had summoned that.

You were a picture perfect portrait I had painted in my mind. On a pedestal of idealism to which I worked to rise. But you ain't want a knight in shining armor, just a vice to hide behind. When I stopped entertaining the distractions you valued most, you opted to drown in spirits rather than give up the ghost. So how ironic that the person you inspired me to become would outgrow you when you were too scared to give sufficient love.

You unknowingly counted on my perpetual stagnation, but I started communicating needs, rebuking his abuses, and held you to your word when you said that you'd have patience. But medicine tasted like poison when you'd only ever ate bullshit. But I say this shit with love, I ain't tryna scream from a pulpit.

Still, I changed the rules when I refused to play the fool. Calling a spade a spade, and your spade was abuse. You found identity in victimhood just how he hoped you would. He taught you love through filters of his narcissism. So when I gave real love, you ain't have the heart to listen. But I've accepted that grief is simply part of 'forgiven.' And self-love is the grievous road known as our deliverance.

–Isaiah Cane

Mom's note on Good, Grief

Isaiah wrote this song during an extremely heartbreaking time; a time where once again, as a mom, I would have preferred to step in and do something to heal his hurt. Fortunately, when Isaiah shared his song with me, I was reminded that God has given Isaiah words to express and process not only his heartache but his life. When he first told me the title, I thought he meant good grief as in, exasperation but then he pointed out the comma between good and grief. Isaiah recognized that he was processing grief and even though it hurt, it was good. With that reminder, *Good, Grief*, I knew Isaiah would be okay.

A Final Word from Isaiah

If you suspect you're autistic, The Ritvo Autism Asperger Diagnostic Scale–Revised (RAADS–R) is a free, online, self-reported questionnaire designed to gauge adult symptoms of autism. Nothing replaces a diagnosis from a psychiatric professional, but the RAADS-R may help ease you into that potential self-discovery.

If you suspect you have OCD, 1) Sorry, I know it's not fun, and 2) the Yale-Brown Obsessive Compulsive Scale is a free, online survey that classifies expressed OCD symptoms by severity and can help simplify the chaotic debilitation often brought on by symptoms. If you achieve a high score, consider help from an OCD specialist trained in Exposure and Response Prevention (ERP).

If you struggle with people-pleasing, codependency, or whatever shade of "I can't be okay if you're not okay" you call it, consider taking Dr. Kristin Neff's online Self-Compassion Survey. It may illuminate areas of your relationship with yourself where you didn't realize you could benefit from growth.

If you suspect you're just trying to make it through the day with everything in order, consider accepting that you're human. Consider that you're literally just trying your best to overcome every obstacle at once while also maintaining your sanity. Consider crying, farting, sleeping—or whatever else in the world you need to do to venture closer to a sense of fulfillment than to one of obligation. And trust me, I'm there with you. At the very least, exhale as if you're flushing out all your tension in one big breath. Did it change anything?

Maybe not. But did you finally do something for yourself? Eh, we're both getting there.

Just because you have obsessive thoughts or perform compulsive behaviors does *not* mean that you have obsessive-compulsive disorder. With OCD, these thoughts and behaviors cause tremendous distress, take up a lot of time (at least one hour per day), and interfere with your daily life and relationships. Most people with obsessive-compulsive disorder have both obsessions and compulsions, but some people experience just one or the other.

Common obsessive thoughts in OCD include:
- Fear of being contaminated by germs or dirt or contaminating others.
- Fear of losing control and harming yourself or others.
- Intrusive sexually explicit or violent thoughts and images.
- Excessive focus on religious or moral ideas.
- Fear of losing or not having things you might need.
- Order and symmetry: the idea that everything must line up "just right."
- Superstitions; excessive attention to something considered lucky or unlucky.

Common compulsive behaviors in OCD include:
- Excessive double-checking of things, such as locks, appliances, and switches.
- Repeatedly checking in on loved ones to make sure they're safe.
- Counting, tapping, repeating certain words, or doing

other senseless things to reduce anxiety.
- Spending a lot of time washing or cleaning.
- Ordering or arranging things "just so."
- Praying excessively or engaging in rituals triggered by religious fear.
- Accumulating "junk" such as old newspapers or empty food containers.

For more information we recommend *The Complete OCD Workbook* by Scott Granet, which includes:

An essential introduction that provides an overview of the primary treatment methods such as CBT, ERP, and mindfulness.

Actionable exercises that use questionnaires, checklists, and reflective prompts to provide a hands-on and personalized approach to treating OCD.

Real stories that offer support throughout your journey to healing, from patients who understand and have overcome struggles associated with OCD.

Available wherever fine books are sold.

For additional OCD information visit: Nathan Peterson Channel *www.youtube.com/@ocdandanxiety/channel*

Acknowledgments

MONICA:

Janie Gallagher for one significant comment she made when my son was just a baby. I had almost forgotten about her words until I started writing this book, then the conversation between us came rushing back. I had confided in Janie that I just wanted to honor God with my desire for writing but was unsure of where it might lead and whether there really was a purpose for writing. I recognize now, over twenty years later, that her simple response that day was actually a prophetic word.

"Who knows sister, maybe God has given you the gift of writing not just for yourself but for writing something with your son one day."

Isaiah Seeing you take accountability for your mental, emotional and spiritual well being, especially only being in your early twenties, has blessed me more than you can imagine. Thank you for your openness with me and for your willingness to share a bit of your journey with others through this book. Thank you for teaching me and Dad about what being on the spectrum is like for you. You know I like to say that I'm your number one fan and that Dad and I are your biggest supporters, but as you've learned about yourself and have openly shared with us, we've learned that you are a fantastic supporter of your mom and dad as well. Thanks for being you, Son.

–Love Mom

Acknowledgments

ISAIAH:

To my NOCD counselor, for turning his personal pain into interpersonal healing.

To my ex-fiancée, who rightfully showed me that I deserved better.

To Isaiah from Isaiah: Listening to my own thoughts without judgment remains the best thing I've done for myself.

About the Authors

Monica Cane is a freelance writer from Northern California. She is the author of *Scrambled Hormones: 60 Days of Encouragement for Moms Raising Teenage Daughters* and *The Lost Coin*.

To learn more about Monica, visit www.monicacane.com

Isaiah Cane draws from his experience on the spectrum for inspiration as a screenwriter in Northern California.

www.ingramcontent.com/pod-product-compliance
Lightning Source LLC
Chambersburg PA
CBHW021640120626
46545CB00002B/632